Managing the Chemically Dependent Nurse

A guide to identification, intervention, and retention

Anne M. Catanzarite, R.N.

AHA books are published by American Hospital Publishing, Inc.,
an American Hospital Association company

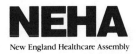
New England Healthcare Assembly

The views expressed in this publication are strictly those of the author and do not necessarily represent official positions of the American Hospital Association.

Library of Congress Cataloging-in-Publication Data

Catanzarite, Anne M.
   Managing the chemically dependent nurse : a guide to identification, intervention, and retention / Anne M. Catanzarite.
             p.   cm.
   Includes bibliographical references.
   ISBN 1-55648-084-9 (pbk.)
   1. Nurses — Substance use. 2. Nurses — Rehabilitation. 3. Nursing services — Personnel management. I. Title.
   [DNLM: 1. Nurses. 2. Professional Impairment. 3. Substance Use Disorders — diagnosis — nurses' instruction. 4. Substance Use Disorders — therapy — nurses' instruction.   WX 270 C3568m]
   RC564.5.N87C38   1992
   362.298'08'8613 — dc20
   DNLM/DLC
   for Library of Congress   92-22053
                                                                       CIP

Catalog no. 154200

©1992 by American Hospital Publishing, Inc.,
an American Hospital Association company

Printed in the USA

𝔸ℍ𝔸 is a service mark of the American Hospital Association used under license by American Hospital Publishing, Inc.

Text set in Trump Medieval
3M — 08/92 — 0322

Audrey Kaufman, Project Editor
Teresa Cappetta-Kroger, Editorial Assistant
Marcia Bottoms, Managing Editor
Peggy DuMais, Production Coordinator
Luke Smith, Cover Designer
Brian Schenk, Books Division Director

To Dolores A. Morgan — nurse, physician, and friend. Her compassion, unwavering commitment, and determined leadership in treating and championing the needs of the chemically dependent have changed the lives of all who know her.

And, to all nurses for their special gift of caring that empowers and renews us all.

Contents

About the Author vi

List of Figures vii

Foreword ix

Preface xi

Acknowledgments xv

Chapter 1. The Disease of Chemical Dependency 1

Chapter 2. Chemical Dependency among Nurses 17

Chapter 3. Signs and Symptoms of Chemical Dependency 29

Chapter 4. Enabling, an Obstacle to Identification
            and Intervention 49

Chapter 5. Documentation of the Signs and Symptoms
            of Chemical Dependency 67

Chapter 6. Preparation for an Intervention 89

Chapter 7. A Sample Intervention 117

Chapter 8. Postintervention and Treatment Issues 133

Chapter 9. Recovery and Return to Practice 159

Chapter 10. A Facilitywide Alcohol and Drug Program 177

Afterword 197

Appendix.   Suggested Resources 201

About the Author

Anne M. Catanzarite, R.N., B.S.N., is nationally recognized for her work with chemically dependent nurses. She has worked in the addiction field for over 16 years, with extensive experience in management and program development. She currently works with health care organizations, regulatory agencies, and professional associations and organizations to provide consultation, training, and program development in the areas of employee assistance, creation of a drug-free workplace, wellness promotion, burnout prevention, and stress management.

Ms. Catanzarite is the former director of Florida's Intervention Project for Nurses, which works to advance the treatment, intervention, and rehabilitation of chemically dependent nurses. She produced, directed, and wrote *Care for the Caregiver*, a videotape on conducting interventions for chemically dependent nurses. Ms. Catanzarite is a featured speaker at national conferences; her special area of interest is facilitating specialized substance abuse programs for nurses and health care institutions. She received her nursing diploma from St. Joseph's Hospital School of Nursing in Syracuse, New York, and her bachelor of science degree from Boston College.

List of Figures

Figure 1-1. Continuum of Drinking Patterns 2

Figure 1-2. Normal Alcohol Metabolism 8

Figure 1-3. Abnormal Alcohol Metabolism 10

Figure 3-1. Checklist of Unsatisfactory Nursing Performance . . 44

Figure 3-2. How an Alcoholic Employee Behaves 46

Figure 4-1. Multiple-System Interactions of the Chemically
Dependent Nurse 51

Figure 4-2. Examples of Attitudes toward Chemical
Dependency 64

Figure 5-1. Controlled Drug Signout Sheet 79

Figure 5-2. Patient George's Medication Record 81

Figure 5-3. Patient George's Nursing Notes 82

Figure 5-4. Controlled Drug Signout Sheet 85

Figure 5-5. Patient Moore's Medication Record 87

Figure 5-6. Patient Taylor's Medication Record 88

Figure 6-1. The 12 Steps of Alcoholics Anonymous 102

Figure 8-1. Sample Treatment Agreement and Releases 136

Figure 8-2. Sample Release of Information to Co-workers 139

Figure 9-1. Sample Return-to-Work Agreement 167

Figure 10-1. Policies and Procedures Governing Employees'
Use of Alcohol or Other Drugs
in the Workplace 179

Figure 10-2. Sample Drug-Testing Policy 187

Foreword

Chemical dependency among nurses is not a new phenomenon. Any student of the history of nursing can find frequent references to the problem of nurses "nipping the bottle" and using narcotics to relieve their own pain and stress. And no wonder—much of a nurse's education points out the benefits of using medications (chemicals) to cure diseases and relieve symptoms. The education of health care workers has little to do with learning how to live a healthy life. In fact, there is a strong tendency in the educational process to highlight rather unhealthy attitudes and behaviors. Physicians are led toward addictive power roles and nurses toward addictive dependency roles. Both directions predispose health care workers to addictions.

The educational orientation of the health profession has also played into one of the foremost symptoms of addiction—denial. The problem goes beyond being "poorly educated" in the area of addictions. Health professionals are actively miseducated. Nurses and physicians are not prepared to deal effectively with chemical dependency. Miseducation coupled with the prevalence of denial results in a transmitted blindness that permeates the consciousness of most health professionals when it comes to understanding the causes, symptoms, and effective treatment of addictions. Not only do they not know the truth about these diseases, but the nature of the educational process (the tendency toward teaching addictive and dependent behaviors in the name of "professionalism") drapes a thick veil of denial over work experiences in these areas.

Managing the Chemically Dependent Nurse lifts that veil and sheds a bright light on the reality of chemical dependency problems in nursing. Anne Catanzarite writes with a clarity that is refreshing about matters that are often shrouded in obtuse language. Of particular value are:

- Checklists that identify early warning signs
- Examples of behavior specific to nursing
- Exercises that survey personal attitudes
- Emphasis on the value of documentation
- Specific instructions for interventions

When I read the section on interventions, I felt nervous and uncomfortable, as I always do when dealing with interventions. This is a profound process that has a profound effect on the lives of all who are involved. The explanation of the process in this book is thorough and clear. The author is an expert, and she provides exemplary guidelines on how to use this powerful process.

The text makes it clear that the responsibility for an intervention rests with the nurse manager who is accountable for the quality of care administered by the members of his or her staff. Most nurse managers would probably prefer not to take responsibility for this activity, but I agree with the author that it is their responsibility. In larger metropolitan communities, professional interventionists are available to act as consultants or to actually manage the intervention process. If a consultant is not available, this book can be used as a guide to achieving a successful intervention. The life of an employee (as well as the lives of others) may be saved by a successful intervention.

One of the greatest assets of this book is the author's use of real-life examples. It is hard to stay in denial while reading about the many true-to-life experiences presented in these pages. In addition, the values of compassion, understanding, and hope permeate the book. The eloquence of the author's passion is evident on every page. This book could only have been written by someone who deeply loves the profession of nursing and who cares about humane treatment for a dread disease.

The conspiracy of silence on chemical dependency that cloaks the profession must be lifted if we are ever to stop unnecessary loss of life to this disease. The statistics do not even begin to tell the story of human resources lost because of denial, misinformation, and fear. This book is important and I am delighted that Catanzarite wrote it.

Marie Manthey, M.N.A., R.N.
President, Creative Nursing Management, Minneapolis
March 1992

Preface

As a nurse manager, have you ever said, "There's something wrong with that nurse. I can't figure it out, but something just isn't right." Or have you wondered, "He's my best nurse. I can't believe he's stealing drugs. How can this be happening?" Or have you asked, "What can I do? I know she's having problems. She's been drinking a lot lately and I can't count on her at work, but I don't know how to deal with her."

Perhaps when a staff nurse returned to work after being treated for chemical dependency, you asked yourself questions like these:

- "Is it safe for him to practice?"
- "Can I ever trust her again?"
- "What do I tell the staff?"
- "What if he starts using again?"
- "Was getting her into treatment worth all the effort?"

If you have faced these questions and concerns, you are not alone. Many managers of chemically dependent nurses express the same concerns, questions, and feelings, and often they remain confused, sad, angry, and frustrated.

All too frequently in the past, the only option managers thought they had after several well-meaning but unsuccessful attempts to help a chemically dependent nurse was to fire him or her. *Managing the Chemically Dependent Nurse: A Guide to Identification, Intervention, and Retention* presents another option—intervention. With intervention, a team of caring colleagues confronts the nurse, persuades the nurse to undergo evaluation and/or treatment, and then supports him or her during recovery and the return-to-work process. It should be stressed that the responsibility of the nurse manager is to identify such problems as inappropriate behavior or impaired practice, not to diagnose the cause of the problem.

The term *chemical dependency* is used throughout this book to describe the disease marked by addiction to, or dependence on, mood-altering substances. This term was chosen over *alcoholism, drug addiction,* and *substance abuse* because it more accurately reflects a dependence on any mood-altering chemicals, including alcohol and other drugs, regardless of whether:

- The nurse is physically dependent on the drug
- The drugs are legal or illegal, pharmaceutical or "street" drugs
- The drugs are prescribed by a physician, bought on the street, obtained from friends, or stolen from the workplace

Throughout the discussion, alcohol is included in references to drugs because its effects are like those of chemicals more commonly labeled "drugs" and can cause even greater devastation in a nurse's life than narcotics or other mood-altering chemicals.

Alcohol and other drugs impair the nurse's professional and personal life. On the job, mood-altering chemicals affect the nurse's:

- Communication skills
- Motor skills
- Work-related knowledge and memory retrieval
- Observation skills

The resulting danger to the chemically dependent nurse's practice is all too apparent. Any delay in effectively intervening can be disastrous for the nurse, his or her patients, and the health care facility.

This book provides nurse managers with the specific knowledge and skills necessary to intervene effectively. Historically, managers have been ill-prepared to identify and intervene with chemically dependent staff members. In addition, health care facilities have not always had the policies and procedures or resources in place to support such efforts.

Managing the Chemically Dependent Nurse was developed as an outgrowth of hundreds of seminars, workshops, and consultations the author conducted with nurses at all administrative, managerial, and staff levels. By learning and consistently applying the principles discussed in this book, nurse managers will be able to:

- Identify nurses who are experiencing problems with drugs and alcohol in the workplace by observing specific signs and symptoms

- Intervene with those nurses and arrange for appropriate treatment and care
- Return recovering nurses to the workplace and effectively monitor their performance
- Establish and implement policies and procedures that will result in consistent management of alcohol and other drug problems in the workplace

Although this book focuses specifically on interventions with staff nurses, the same procedures apply to all nurses at all levels, as well as to other health care workers. If your health care facility does not have an employee assistance program (EAP) in place to help chemically dependent employees, this guide outlines the procedures to take when that responsibility lies with the nurse manager or nurse executive. If your facility has an EAP, the same procedures apply, although responsibilities for carrying them out may vary. In either situation, it is essential that the nurse manager be actively involved in the intervention process for nurses on his or her unit.

Also addressed in this book is the new legislation protecting recovering chemically dependent employees. The Americans with Disabilities Act (ADA) became effective July 26, 1992, for all private employers including nonfederal health care facilities with more than 25 employees; employers with 15 to 24 employees will be affected as of July 26, 1994.

The ADA protects employees and applicants for employment who are "qualified individuals with disabilities" from discrimination in the areas of job application, hiring, advancement, discharge, compensation, and training. The ADA protects alcoholics and recovering drug users who do not currently engage in the illegal use of drugs and who either have been successfully rehabilitated or are participating in a supervised rehabilitation program.

One specific area of concern to nurse managers is in providing "reasonable accommodation" for the recovering nurse. The specific effects of the ADA as they apply to the content of this book are identified throughout. However, legal counsel should be sought in the development of the health care facility's specific policies and procedures.

It is also significant to note that the Board of Trustees of the American Hospital Association recently approved a policy that strongly encourages health care facilities to adopt written substance abuse policies, including provisions for drug and alcohol testing. The policy suggests that it is imperative for health care institutions to conduct educational programs for employees. The AHA believes that without appropriate employee education, treatment, and rehabilitation, the benefits of implementing a testing policy cannot be fully realized.

Once managers start using the skills acquired from reading this book, they will reap the rewards of effective intervention and positive resolution of a complicated management problem. One reward is greater confidence in their own personal and managerial skills. Another is the win–win situation they create by helping chemically dependent nurses on their staffs. The health care facility wins because it reduces its liability and retains qualified, experienced nurses; the nurses win because their jobs, lives, and careers are saved.

As one recovering nurse so eloquently stated:

Intervention saved my life. My addiction had become so great that I was immobilized. I couldn't ask for help. I felt hopeless. I couldn't initiate any change.

I'm forever grateful to my supervisor for confronting me with my addiction and getting me into treatment. If she had not intervened, I would probably be dead today.

Acknowledgments

The act of writing is a singular activity. I sat by myself as I put ideas, thoughts, and experience into written form. Yet I was not alone. This book and the process outlined within it could not have been developed without the ongoing commitment, support, and input of many very special people. Although it is not possible to mention everyone, the following people must be acknowledged.

All the nurses I have had the opportunity to know through my work, who have supported the movement to responsibly care for nurses and who have shared their concerns with me. I recognize their individual and collective contributions. They are nurse managers, staff nurses, nurse administrators and directors, and staff members of alternative programs who have honestly and openly confronted the difficult issues in a manner that has changed the way we look at caring for each other. They include Daryl Devota, Doug Arrington, Charlotte Preston-Santa, Melinda Hardie, Ann Rudolph, Arie Keys, Sharon Douglas, Evelyn Polk, Roger Brown, Sue Vial, Joy Fitzpatrick, Nena Novik, Fran Haddock, Karen Scipio-Skinner, Gaurdia Bannister, Connee Riley, Lee Talbot, Don Gramling, Carolyn Vallone, Marie Manthey, Pam Erb, Judy Willis, Paula Massey, Joyce Dorner, Linda Crosby, Etta Williams, Pat Green, Nancy Miller, Nancy Breen, Jeanne Stark, Natalia Cruz, Betty Taylor, and Nancy Payne.

Many others, including employee assistance counselors, human resource personnel, regulatory personnel, treatment counselors, and administrators, have made a real difference in the care nurses receive: Sy Sokatch, Ingrid Ciucivitch, Joni Kennedy, Bob Hinds, Jim Hall, John Kelly, Jennifer Deloach, Sheila Dunn, R. C. Miller, Mary MacDowell, Lisa Bassett, and Bill Furlow.

Judy Ritter, director of the Florida Board of Nursing, offered me the opportunity to direct the Intervention Project for Nurses. Her insight, humor, willingness to share expertise and knowledge, and ongoing friendship facilitated my work and contributed greatly to this book. Jean Sullivan, director of the Washington Health Professionals Services, blazed a trail for many of us to follow in providing care and services for chemically dependent nurses. Discovery, the program she founded in California to assist nurses, reinforced the reality that as nurses we can and must effectively care for each other. Linda Smith, current director of the Intervention Project for Nurses, provides continued leadership in assisting the chemically dependent nurse. Dolores A. Morgan, physician and addictionist, has continued to inspire me because of her commitment to ensuring the highest level of uncompromised care for addicts and alcoholics. She has treated hundreds of nurses with a combination of skill, knowledge, tough love, and dedication.

Audrey Kaufman, product line manager at American Hospital Publishing, is gratefully acknowledged for her continued support, encouragement, and patience with this first-time author. She has performed above and beyond the call of duty. Liz Kramer, editor with the New England Healthcare Assembly, enthusiastically responded to my proposal for this book and worked with AHPI to see it take form. Janet Plant, editor and writer, patiently directed me in transforming my thoughts into manuscript form.

Rhonda Rhodes, senior counsel for the American Hospital Association, provided a thorough legal review of the manuscript to ensure that it provides appropriate and up-to-date guidance on current legislation, particularly the Americans with Disabilities Act.

My parents, Frank and Patricia Catanzarite, constantly encouraged my efforts; my brothers and their wives, Paul and Sharon, Frank and Carol, welcomed me into their homes and provided an atmosphere of support and encouragement that allowed me to continue to work on the manuscript; and my sisters, Cathy Medina and Louise Caster, are acknowledged for always being there.

Finally, and most important, my daughter Rachel, whose unconditional love, patience, and understanding were always there, especially when I needed to work to meet deadlines.

The Disease of Chemical Dependency

One author who works in the chemical dependency field described how it feels to be chemically dependent in the following way:

> To be chemically dependent is to feel sick and tired most of the time. It is to know deep down that you're stuck feeling this way unless you can get your hands on a drink, a pill, a fix, a joint, a snort. It is to know deep down that you're a prisoner.[1]

Why do people, including nurses, use psychoactive chemicals such as alcohol, narcotics, tranquilizers, and other mind-altering and mood-altering substances? The answer they give can be as simple as one of the following:

- "It's a social occasion."
- "A drink after work helps me relax."
- "I like the way it makes me feel."
- "I want to be happy, not depressed."
- "It's a family tradition."

Or as complicated as one of these:

- "It makes me feel normal."
- "I need to."
- "I can't get through the day without it."

Not everyone who uses a potentially addictive drug actually becomes dependent on it. For example, only about 10 percent of those who drink become addicted to alcohol.[2] As nurses, we are also aware that some patients become addicted to prescribed medications while most other patients do not. The initial drug use was legal and medically warranted in such cases, but the result was still addiction for vulnerable individuals. Why do some people become addicted when the majority do not? Is it a genetic predisposition or some other factor?

This chapter attempts to answer these questions and acquaint nurse managers with some basic information on chemical dependency. Specifically, chapter 1 covers the following subjects:

- *The basic patterns of alcohol and other drug use:* Addiction progresses through predictable stages. A good understanding of this progression can help managers to identify addictive tendencies among staff members as early as possible.
- *Chemical dependency as a disease:* Chemical dependency meets all the criteria to be considered a disease.
- *Predisposing factors:* There is no definitive explanation of why some people become addicted and others do not. There are, however, a number of physiological differences between alcoholics and nonalcoholics that may explain the alcoholic's vulnerability to alcohol addiction and may indicate the etiology of other forms of chemical dependency as well.

Stages of Chemical Dependency

The best way to understand chemical dependency is to look at it as falling on a continuum from occasional use to addiction. To date, most of the research and work with addictive substances has been done in the area of alcohol abuse. In fact, alcohol is the most widely used psychoactive drug. We will therefore use alcohol to illustrate patterns of use and the progression to addiction. (See figure 1-1.) Experts in the field of chemical dependency agree that the patterns and progression are very similar, whether the chemical involved is alcohol, narcotics, or some other addictive substance.

Figure 1-1. Continuum of Drinking Patterns

Abstinence	(1) Nonproblem, Nondependent	(2) Problem, Heavy	(3) Problem, Dependent
No drinking at all	Social drinking	Stress drinking	Addiction
		Abusive drinking	Chemical dependency

Patterns of Progression to Addiction

The initial drinking pattern is commonly called *social drinking.* Social drinkers use alcohol primarily to enhance already-pleasant experiences in social situations. They drink for relaxation and entertainment. Also included in this category are individuals for whom drinking is a ritual: a glass of wine or beer with a meal, for example, or wine as part of a religious celebration or event. Other social drinkers may enjoy a cold beer on a hot day or a mixed drink after work.

Social drinkers share some common characteristics:

- They usually drink small amounts of alcohol.
- They do not experience any harmful side effects, such as loss of control or impaired judgment.
- They feel that alcohol generates a generally positive feeling.
- They do not need to consume alcohol to have a good time.
- They are still in control; they make conscious decisions about when to use alcohol.
- They follow social rules and laws about alcohol use, including when, where, and how much.

Getting drunk is a rare or accidental occurrence at this stage. There is no emotional cost to drinking or any violation of personal values.

The second drinking pattern in the progression to alcoholism is *problem or heavy drinking.* Typically, heavy drinkers live in a persistent high-stress state and use alcohol to relieve the stress. Others may use alcohol intermittently when stress levels are high and cut down when stress levels are low. For the problem drinker, there is usually no demonstrable crisis causing the stress. Instead, problems and stresses are pervasive and are not related to any particular event. Problem drinkers "drink in order to escape their problems and to reduce the mental pain associated with these problems."[3]

Some common characteristics of heavy and problem drinkers include the following:

- They usually drink large amounts of alcohol.
- They usually drink to the point of intoxication. However, they also have periods of sobriety.
- They suffer the negative side effects of alcohol use (such as loss of control, impaired judgment, family and work problems) with increasing frequency.
- They show diminished concern about the effect their drinking has on their behavior.

- They break social or legal drinking rules and violate their own values.
- They sometimes experience painful feelings of guilt or remorse.
- They often use alcohol to lessen their emotional pain.
- They experience an important relationship with alcohol.
- They become defensive about their drinking and find the need to justify or rationalize it.

These adverse effects may occur after a single drinking episode or persistent heavy use.

The third pattern of drinking is *dependent drinking.* Dependent drinkers, who are physically and/or psychologically addicted to alcohol, experience many negative consequences of alcohol use at this point:

- They experience the harmful side effects of alcohol use almost every time they drink.
- They experience negative feelings, such as shame, guilt, and low self-esteem.
- They begin to lose their ability to function emotionally, socially, spiritually, intellectually, and physically.
- They lose control over their use of alcohol, becoming obsessed and preoccupied with it.
- They delude themselves into thinking that they function normally while intoxicated.
- They refuse to believe other people's accounts of their uncharacteristic behavior under the influence of alcohol.

At this point, the person is chemically dependent and caught in the cycle of addiction. It is important to realize, however, that the problem or heavy drinker (pattern two) does not automatically progress to stage three. As mentioned earlier, only 10 percent of alcohol users actually become addicted.

The alcoholic's progression through these three patterns can take place over a number of years. The typical progression for those who use drugs other than alcohol is generally the same, although the time from initial use to addiction is generally measured in weeks and months rather than in years. Heroin or morphine use, for example, can result in addiction in just four weeks.[4]

A Four-Stage Model

Vernon Johnson, D.D., a founder of the Johnson Institute in Minneapolis, developed a four-stage model of progression to addiction.[5]

The Johnson Institute is well known for its research and educational activities in the field of chemical dependency.

Stage One

Johnson refers to the first stage of addiction as *learning the mood swing.* This is the first step for everyone who takes a mood-altering chemical. The chemical usually is taken for recreational or medicinal use, and the experience is generally pleasant. People become aware of the substance's positive effect, usually a feeling of relaxation, and experience no adverse side effects. With alcohol, if they drink too much or too fast and get sick, they are usually able to modify their drinking behavior so that the next episode will be pleasant and predictable.

Stage Two

Stage two of Johnson's progression is called *seeking the mood swing.* For example, individuals who have learned the effects of alcohol or another drug will use the substance again when they want to achieve the same feeling. At times, they may overdo it, but in general they experience no significant adverse effects. Many people who drink alcohol or use other drugs remain at this stage, never progressing to stage three.

Stage Three

The third stage is called *harmful dependency.* At this stage, users may begin to lose control and experience the adverse effects of alcohol or other drug use. Friends and employers may complain about their behavior. Socially accepted rules of consumption are broken. More money is spent on alcohol or drugs than users intend or can afford. They begin to feel that alcohol or drug use is not as much fun as it used to be.

Stage Four

In the fourth stage, *using to feel normal,* drinkers or drug users have lost the ability to control their alcohol or other drug use. They drink or use drugs to feel normal, to avoid the pain of withdrawal. They drink or consume drugs compulsively, and their primary focus is on obtaining their supplies of alcohol or other drugs. They begin to experience the physical problems that result from chronic intoxication and blackouts. When others confront them about their behavior, they deny that they have a problem. By this stage, they are firmly entrenched in the cycle of addiction.

Chemical Dependency as a Disease

Most people, including nurses, react with disbelief and shock when confronted with the reality that nurses can be addicts and alcoholics. Many people believe that nurses are above such problems and that health care professionals are somehow immune to chemical dependency. This attitude is often based on the erroneous belief that chemical dependency is a moral weakness rather than a disease.

Chemical dependency is classified as a disease, not as a condition or disorder. It meets all the criteria of a disease: it has predictable symptoms, it is primary, it is progressive, it is chronic, and it can be fatal if left untreated.

A Primary Disease

Chemical dependency is not secondary to any other disease, nor is it the direct result of an emotional condition. In fact, chemical dependency itself causes physical and emotional problems and can aggravate already-existing medical conditions. In *The 350 Secondary Diseases/Disorders to Alcoholism*, for example, Toby Rice Drews presents a comprehensive list of the medical consequences, both physical and psychological, that are secondary to alcoholism.[6] Overall, an estimated 25 to 50 percent of all admissions to general hospitals and psychiatric hospitals can be linked to some type of alcohol involvement.[7]

A Progressive Disease

Chemical dependency runs a predictable course. Without treatment, the addicted person's disease gets worse, and the deterioration in all aspects of his or her life — physical, intellectual, social, and emotional — advances. Without treatment, chemical dependency gets worse.

A Chronic Disease

The disease is chronic and permanent. Once people become chemically dependent, they remain chemically dependent for the rest of their lives. The disease can, however, be treated and arrested. Very often its medical consequences can be reversed, especially when the disease is treated in its early stages. Chemically dependent people can live happy, productive lives as long as they abstain from using mood-altering chemicals.

As with other chronic diseases, relapse is always possible. The most effective ongoing recoveries have been achieved through treatment and recovery programs that include abstinence. Abstinence is an obstacle for some alcohol- and addiction-prone persons who believe that they can control their alcohol or drug use through willpower. Most attempts to "learn" how to drink moderately have failed, however. Relapses have also occurred when recovering alcoholics or addicts were placed on tranquilizers or other mood-altering drugs under a physician's prescription. The usual result is that they became addicted to the new drugs; this phenomenon is called *cross-addiction*. Reports of recovering alcoholics and addicts who have relapsed as a result of using over-the-counter cough medicines are not unusual. Such relapses may progress to the full-blown, active stages of chemical dependency. Therefore, chemically dependent people must abstain totally from all mood-altering chemicals. Even when analgesics are required after a surgical procedure, they should be prescribed only by a physician who is experienced in treating addictions.

A Potentially Fatal Disease

When chemical dependency is not arrested, it can eventually prove fatal. Addicted nurses, like others with the disease, usually die prematurely. Insurance companies report that active alcoholics have a life span that is 12 years shorter than that of nonalcoholics.[8]

In the case of alcoholics, the cause of death may be any of the following:[9]

- *Accidental:* Alcohol is a factor in the leading causes of accidental deaths in the United States, including traffic accidents, falls, and fires. For instance, in 1987, 40 percent of automobile accident fatalities involved at least one driver who was legally intoxicated.
- *Physical:* Death from cirrhosis of the liver, which is usually caused by heavy alcohol use, was the ninth-leading cause of death in the United States in 1986. Bleeding ulcers, esophageal and gastric cancers, and cardiovascular diseases have also been linked to alcoholism.
- *Emotional:* Twenty to 36 percent of suicide victims have a history of alcohol abuse or were drinking shortly before their deaths. Usually, suicides involving alcohol are impulsive rather than premeditated.

Research reported in the next section points to some of the physiological factors that predispose individuals to the disease of chemical dependency.

Predisposing Factors

Why do only 10 percent of all drinkers become alcoholics? Why do some patients "get hooked" on prescription drugs? No definitive answers have been discovered to date. However, scientists have been able to identify a number of physiological differences between alcoholics and non-alcoholics that may explain alcoholics' vulnerability to alcohol addiction. So far, most of the research into predisposing factors has focused on alcoholism rather than on other drug addictions. This section summarizes that research.

Abnormal Metabolism of Alcohol

Alcohol is metabolized differently in alcoholics than it is in nonalcoholics. To understand abnormal metabolism in alcoholics, it is essential to first understand how alcohol is metabolized normally in nonalcoholics.

After alcohol enters the bloodstream of a nonalcoholic, it is chemically metabolized in the liver by two enzymes. The process breaks alcohol down into carbon dioxide and water, both of which are eliminated from the body through perspiration, urine, and breath. (See figure 1-2.)

Figure 1-2. Normal Alcohol Metabolism

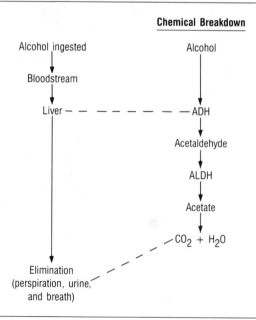

The two crucial liver enzymes are alcohol dehydrogenase (ADH) and acetaldehyde dehydrogenase (ALDH). First, ADH converts alcohol to acetaldehyde. Then ALDH converts acetaldehyde to acetate. Acetate is subsequently broken down into carbon dioxide and water.

A normally functioning liver can metabolize half an ounce of alcohol in an hour. When alcohol is ingested in large quantities, however, the liver must speed up the rate of metabolism. In the process, it is often overtaxed and cannot convert acetaldehyde to acetate. Levels of acetaldehyde, which is a toxic substance, build up in the bloodstream. As they do, the nonalcoholic drinker suffers dizziness, nausea, rapid heartbeat, mental confusion, and eventually a hangover.

High acetaldehyde levels damage liver cells, and persistently high levels over a long period of time cause permanent cell damage. Acetaldehyde also interferes with the functioning of other organs. It inhibits protein synthesis in heart muscle, for instance, and causes bizarre and complex chemical reactions in the brain.[10]

Alcoholics metabolize alcohol differently than nonalcoholics in three ways:[11]

- Acetaldehyde is present in higher amounts.
- Tetrahydroisoquinolines (TIQs), highly addictive neurochemicals similar to morphine, are present — usually in large amounts — in alcoholics, but TIQs are not manufactured in any sizable amount in nonalcoholic social or heavy drinkers. Many researchers believe that TIQs are the root cause of addiction.
- The alcoholic's brain cell membranes are abnormally thickened and require a constant supply of alcohol for the person to feel "normal." When alcohol is withheld, the membranes function poorly and the alcoholic experiences discomfort and withdrawal symptoms.

In the alcoholic, liver enzyme abnormalities prevent the normal metabolism of alcohol. Acetaldehyde builds up, is transported to the brain, passes through the blood–brain barrier, and disrupts the chemical balance of the brain cells. Although the blood–brain barrier protects brain cells from most other toxins, acetaldehyde can permeate it easily.

Once in the brain, acetaldehyde combines with neurotransmitters to produce TIQs. In turn, TIQs attach themselves to certain neuroreceptors to produce a feeling of well-being, which continues as long as the person continues to drink. By this time, the brain cells have become addicted and crave alcohol. The effect on the brain is similar to that of heroin: the brain feels good, wants more, and needs more. (See figure 1-3.)

Figure 1-3. Abnormal Alcohol Metabolism

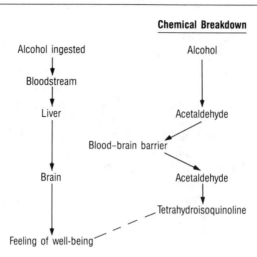

To date, no tests have been developed to screen patients for ADH and ALDH abnormalities or for TIQ levels. Research continues in these areas. One day, tests may enable health care professionals to alert people to their potential for alcoholism before the disease develops.

Other Biochemical Differences

Other research provides additional insight into the causes of alcoholism, as well as the complex nature and biochemistry of the disease. K. Blum and M. Trachtenberg[12] have summarized the results of many scientific experiments, both animal and human studies, conducted in the past few decades. These experiments have led to seeing "alcoholism in its true light: a deficiency disease, often genetic in origin, involving the 'neurotransmitters' that act as messengers between brain neurons" (p. 33). The following discoveries, summarized by Blum and Trachtenberg, are significant in understanding this complex disease.

Opiate receptor sites have been discovered in certain areas of neurons in brain cells. These naturally occurring sites are present in all individuals, and their function is to receive opiate molecules. This discovery led scientists to the additional discovery of endorphins, naturally produced chemical substances in the brain. Endorphins were labeled "opioids" because of their morphinelike nature and their tendency to reduce pain and stress, increase immune system functioning, and produce feelings of well-being and euphoria. The endorphins, or opioids, attach themselves naturally to the opiate receptor sites.

Most people are familiar with the term "runner's high," the feeling achieved through rigorous physical activity. It has been attributed to the increased production of endorphins after activity and exercise. Another example of the effects of endorphins has been seen in persons suffering from arthritis. Their pain often decreases with physical activity, as endorphins attach themselves to the neurons. The endorphins contain various amino acids, including enkephalins. Under normal conditions, enkephalins attach themselves to opiate receptor sites, producing feelings of well-being as well as pain relief and stress reduction.

In the nonalcoholic, endorphins, including enkephalins, are present in high quantities and freely move across the synapse, attach to receptor sites, and produce a general feeling of well-being. In the genetic alcoholic, who is believed to have been born with a deficiency of internal opioids, the synthesis of endorphins and enkephalins is low, and the experience is much different. Very few of the internal opioids are released and reach the receptors. "As a result, the individual has a feeling of incompleteness, of craving. This situation also may apply to children of alcoholics."[13]

The preceding section of this chapter showed how abnormal metabolism of alcohol by an alcoholic (figure 1-3) produces an increased level of acetaldehyde that, combined with the neurotransmitters, produces tetrahydroisoquinolines (TIQs), the morphinelike substances that interfere with the binding of enkephalins to the opiate receptor sites. The TIQs themselves occupy the receptor sites, producing a feeling of well-being—false as it may be. Once the euphoria passes, more alcohol must be ingested to maintain the feeling and prevent negative side effects, and the cycle of addiction continues.

Furthermore, when TIQs fill the receptor sites and a feeling of well-being or euphoria is generated, the internal message sent to the cells is that enough opioids are available. This message causes a decrease in internal opioid (endorphin) production. As a result, the person needs more alcohol to feel normal and becomes dependent on alcohol.

On the basis of various studies, Blum and Trachtenberg have theorized that a deficiency in opioid activity in the central nervous system may determine the difference between alcohol-preferring and non-alcohol-preferring animals. Those with lower endorphin levels seek out alcohol. Human studies have shown that normal social drinkers have high endorphin levels, but alcoholics have significantly reduced levels. Additional studies have also found that "stress, low enkephalin levels, and alcohol preference appeared closely related."[14]

11

The results of the experiments summarized by Blum and Trachtenberg are important because they clarify the difference in brain chemistry between the alcoholic and the nonalcoholic. These findings have generated additional research aimed at developing non–habit-forming methods to correct neurotransmitter and endorphin deficiencies, whether genetic or environmental in origin.

Heredity

Throughout history, it has been observed that alcoholism runs in families; the actual cause for the hereditary link, however, was not identified until recently. In the past, many people believed that somehow children raised in alcoholic homes learned the behavior, inherited a weakness in moral fiber, or were just lacking in willpower. Recent research has confirmed that alcoholism is indeed hereditary but that it is transmitted genetically through body chemistry, rather than environmentally.

The hereditary nature of alcoholism has been confirmed by numerous studies. In 1979, N. S. Cotton reviewed 39 familial alcoholism studies published over a 10-year period. Among her findings were these:[15]

- An alcoholic is more likely than a nonalcoholic to have an alcoholic parent or other relative.
- In two-thirds of the studies, at least 25 percent of alcoholics had alcoholic fathers.
- Most of the studies found high rates of alcoholism among parents of alcoholics. Several also found high rates among siblings.
- Fathers and brothers of alcoholics were more likely to have problems with alcohol than were mothers and sisters.
- Many studies indicated that a major risk factor for developing alcoholism is being the close relative of an alcoholic.

Based on her review, Cotton estimated that on average one-third of any sample of alcoholics will have had at least one parent who was an alcoholic.

Research conducted by D. W. Goodwin, M.D., a psychiatrist, reinforced the link between alcoholism and heredity. In general, his studies indicate that children of alcoholics face a much higher risk of alcoholism themselves. In a study of 30-year-old Danish males who were adopted at six weeks of age by nonalcoholic families, Goodwin found that boys who had alcoholic natural fathers were three times more likely to become alcoholics than were boys who had nonalcoholic natural fathers. The sons of alcoholic fathers also became alcoholics at an earlier age.[16]

Psychiatric problems proved not to be a relevant factor in the development of alcoholism, according to Goodwin's study. There were no differences between the sons of alcoholic and nonalcoholic natural fathers with regard to the incidence of depression, anxiety neuroses, personality disturbances, or other psychiatric conditions.[17]

In another study, Goodwin compared two categories of sons of alcoholics: (1) those raised by an alcoholic parent and (2) those raised by an adoptive nonalcoholic family. Sons raised in the nonalcoholic environment were just as likely to develop alcoholism as those raised by an alcoholic natural parent.[18]

In a 1983 study, G. Vaillant further confirmed the familial link in the development of alcoholism. He found that the consistent factor in predicting alcoholism was an individual's having had an alcoholic parent. His conclusions, based on longitudinal studies spanning 40 years, included the following:[19]

- Boys with alcoholic parents were five times more likely to develop alcoholism than boys with nonalcoholic parents.
- The alcoholism trait can be passed on from mother or father to son or daughter and from grandparent to grandchild. Although it may appear that alcoholism can skip a generation, in reality, the trait is present but may not be manifested in individuals who do not drink. Such individuals, nonetheless, carry the trait and pass it on to future generations.

Scientists now generally agree that the predisposition for alcoholism is transmitted genetically through biochemistry, not through the mind or the environment.[20] It occurs in all groups, regardless of race, sex, profession, or social status. However, environmental factors can also play a role in the development of chemical dependency. High levels of stress, ineffective coping skills, and lack of education regarding chemical dependency may increase the likelihood that people will use psychoactive drugs to cope with reality. However, of people who use drugs to cope, those with a family history of the disease will have a greater risk for becoming addicted than those without such a family history.

Therefore, a number of factors contribute to the development of alcoholism. The greatest risks are having a close relative who is an alcoholic and inheriting the biochemistry that predisposes an individual to the disease. According to one report:

The scientific evidence clearly indicates an interplay of various hereditary, physiological factors—metabolic, hormonal, and neurological—which work together in tandem to determine the individual's susceptibility to alcoholism. . . . Yet, while additional predisposing factors to alcoholism will undoubtedly be discovered, abundant knowledge already exists to confirm that alcoholism is a hereditary, physiological disease and to account fully for its onset and progression.[21]

Summary

People who are chemically dependent become addicted to psychoactive, or mood-altering, drugs. Common addictive drugs include alcohol, narcotics, and tranquilizers.

On the road to addiction, chemically dependent individuals pass through various stages, each with its own characteristic signs and symptoms. People who drink alcohol or use other drugs but do not become physically addicted can also pass through some of the same stages. However, they stop short of physical addiction.

The reasons why some people become addicted and others do not appear to be physiological and genetic. Research into alcoholism shows that alcohol metabolism in the liver differs between the two groups. Alcoholics also seem to have lower levels of endorphins (morphine-like substances in the brain) and tend to crave alcohol as a result. Thus, the liver and brain chemistry differs between alcoholics and non-alcoholics. Alcoholism and other chemical dependencies are *not* learned behaviors, with children mimicking their parents, as was once thought.

Researchers have determined and health care professionals are beginning to realize that chemical dependency is a primary disease. Its characteristic signs and symptoms include loss of control and predictability, compulsive use, and continued use despite adverse consequences. The disease is chronic and progressive, and it can be fatal. It can, however, be successfully treated.

☐ *References*

1. Leite, E. *How It Feels to Be Chemically Dependent.* Minneapolis: Johnson Institute, 1987.
2. Milan, J. R., and Ketcham, K. *Under the Influence.* Seattle: Madrona Publishers, 1981, p. 26.
3. Mann, G. A. *Recovery of Reality.* San Francisco: Harper and Row Publishers, 1979.
4. Milan and Ketcham.
5. Johnson, V. *Intervention: How to Help Someone Who Doesn't Want Help.* Minneapolis: Johnson Institute, 1986.

6. Drews, T. R. *The 350 Secondary Disorders/Diseases to Alcoholism.* South Plainfield, NJ: Bridge Publishing, 1985.

7. Johnson.

8. Johnson.

9. Secretary of Health and Human Services. *Alcohol and Health, Seventh Special Report to the U.S. Congress.* Washington, DC: U.S. Government Printing Office, 1990.

10. Milan and Ketcham.

11. Fitzgerald, K. W. *Alcoholism: The Genetic Inheritance.* New York City: Doubleday, 1988.

12. Blum, K., and Trachtenberg, M. New insights into the causes of alcoholism. *Professional Counselor* 1(5):33–36, 1987.

13. Blum and Trachtenberg, p. 35.

14. Blum and Trachtenberg, p. 34.

15. Cotton, N. S. The familial incidence of alcoholism: a review. *Journal of Studies on Alcohol* 40(1):89–116, 1979.

16. Goodwin, D. W., Schulsinger, F., Hermansen, L., Guze, S. B., and Winokur, G. Alcohol problems in adoptees raised apart from biological parents. *Archives of General Psychiatry* 28:238–43, Feb. 1973.

17. Goodwin and others.

18. Goodwin, D. W., Schulsinger, F., Moller, N., Hermansen, L., Winokur, G., and Guze, S. Drinking problems in adopted and non-adopted sons of alcoholics. *Archives of General Psychiatry* 31:164–69, Aug. 1974.

19. Vaillant, G. *The Natural History of Alcoholism: Causes, Patterns, and Paths to Recovery.* Cambridge, MA: Harvard University Press, 1983.

20. Johnson.

21. Mann.

Chemical Dependency among Nurses

The tragedy of chemical dependency among nurses can best be illustrated by a real-life example. All the names used in the case histories throughout this book have been changed to protect the nurses' real identities.

A Real Story

The call came into the Intervention Project for Nurses (IPN) office at 2:30 p.m., from a woman who identified herself as "Sharon, a nurse." She was sobbing as she told Jean, an IPN staff member, why she was calling.

Sharon had been working at University Hospital through the Home Health Agency for the previous two weeks. Yesterday, when she reported for duty on the night shift, she was told to go home because she was in no condition to work. She was also told that she would be reported to the agency and that she would never be allowed to work at the hospital again.

The supervisor at the hospital reported to the Home Health Agency that Sharon had arrived one hour late, had been rude to the staff, and had smelled of alcohol. In a phone conversation later that night, the agency director asked Sharon to report to the office the next morning at 10:00 a.m.

Sharon admitted to Jean that she had had a few drinks before going to work the night before but hadn't thought that it would be a problem. She had often reported for work after consuming alcohol in the past, and no one had ever said anything. She also admitted that she didn't believe she could have made it to work without those drinks.

When Sharon arrived at the agency office that morning, Martha, the agency's director, told her that she could no longer work for the agency. She was paid for the three days she had worked that week. Martha instructed Sharon to call the Intervention Project for Nurses herself or she would have to report her to the Board of Nursing for disciplinary action.

When Sharon left the office, she was distraught and had no idea what to do. Because she did not own a car, she walked the four miles home — home for the past two months had been a run-down motel, the kind of place usually referred to as a "flophouse." She shared a small room with her two children, ages six and seven. For the past year, she had been working through agencies and moving from motel to motel with her kids, always looking for a cheaper place to stay. When Sharon worked, the children stayed alone in the motel.

On the telephone that afternoon, Sharon cried and sounded suicidal. However, Jean was able to keep her on the phone while another staff member contacted two recovering nurses who lived in the same area as Sharon.

Sharon continued talking with Jean from a pay phone outside the motel in the pouring rain. She told Jean that her life had started to "unravel" about six years ago. She described a history that included problems with her work and her health. She admitted using alcohol and other drugs. Her husband had left her and the children three years ago and did nothing to support them financially. She had lost touch with her family, who lived in another part of the country, and at this point in her life, it was difficult to see any way out or to have any hope.

Sharon felt desperate, without hope, and she was concerned for her children. It was obvious to Jean that immediate action was required. While Jean continued to talk with Sharon, the two recovering nurses arrived at the motel, found Sharon, and immediately began to help her.

There is much more to the story, but the most important detail is that Sharon is alive and recovering today. She shares her story with other nurses to provide hope and, even more important, to explain the necessity of nurses caring for and intervening with other nurses.

Sharon had gone from being a highly respected and competent head nurse in a neurological intensive care unit to being demoted several times and finally becoming suicidal. The deterioration in her career and her personal and professional relationships was directly related to her advancing chemical dependency. Had somebody intervened earlier, she might not have reached the crisis level. And, had she not made that call, with the resulting response and intervention, she might be dead today. Sharon is convinced that she would have been.

Sharon and Jean are real people. The story is true, and unfortunately, it's not an unusual story. It has happened many times, in many different ways, to many different nurses. The setting may be different, the specific events may change, but the story is the same—a competent, caring nurse deteriorates while her colleagues look on helplessly. She works in a highly sophisticated system that provides the most advanced medical care, compassionately caring for those who are ill. Yet, all too often, her own treatable disease goes unnoticed.

The reality today is that most nurses know someone who is chemically dependent. The good news is that many nurses are intervening to interrupt the cycle of addiction among their co-workers.

The story of Sharon and other nurses like her is important to tell and retell for many reasons. First, there was a happy ending for Sharon. She received treatment and her life was restored. Second, Sharon's story clearly shows how people who care and know what to do can make a difference. That is the essence of this book—to provide hope and knowledge that empower nurse managers to intervene with chemically dependent nurses.

Chapter 1 dealt with the disease of chemical dependency in general, the basic stages and some of the known risk factors. The rest of this chapter will address the specific impact that chemical dependency has on nurses. It provides an historical look at addiction among nurses, risk factors specific to nurses, the prevalence of addiction among nurses, and the costs of chemical dependency to individuals and health care employers.

Historical Perspective

Chemical dependency among nurses is nothing new. It was noted in the health care literature of the early 1900s. Only in the past few decades, however, have nursing administrators, state boards of nursing, and educators recognized that the use of alcohol and other drugs by nurses has a significant impact on nursing practice. The recent attention to this issue in the nursing field in some ways parallels the country's reaction to alcohol and other drug problems in the general population. Although it has not been proved that health care professionals have a greater risk for addiction than does the general population, the consequences may be greater because of the work they do.

Soon after the turn of the century, substance abuse was recognized as a problem confronting nurses. No consistent or specific effort was made to combat the problem at that time, but at least there was an awareness of the special vulnerability of nurses to addiction. The most definitive acknowledgment of the problem came from physicians, who were usually responsible for the training of nurses in the early 20th century.[1] At that time, nursing education included instruction in morality and ethics. Nurses were warned through their professional journal

of their moral and legal responsibilities in the prescription and purchase of medications. Nurses were prohibited by law from prescribing
but could legally purchase narcotics such as morphine and cocaine.
Hyson warned nurses of the increasing incidence of uncontrollable
habits with respect to using these drugs.[2] He did not indicate that
nurses were a high-risk group for addiction or that they self-prescribed
the narcotics. However, he did mention that nurses viewed these medications as a "cure-all." He also stated, "It seems incredible that a nurse,
an intelligent trained nurse, would to any degree take part in anything
like this; that they do, only proves that they are human."[3]

The need for nurses to be strong and well in body and mind was
a common theme in the nursing literature of the early 1900s. It was
frequently suggested that the nurse needed to appear invulnerable. The
suggestion that a nurse might fall victim to addiction was considered
farfetched among the general population and nurses alike.[4]

Another early reference to addiction among nurses came in 1915
in an article written by physician C. V. Pearson,[5] who discussed the
incidence of self-prescribed morphine use by nurses. Some of the reasons he cited for the prevalence of "morphinism" among nurses (as well
as among physicians, dentists, and pharmacists) were the addictive
nature of morphine and the lack of proper education and preparation
of physicians and nurses for handling such drugs. "The nurse has all
the dangers of becoming an addict that laity have," Pearson explained,
"and in addition to these dangers, the danger of easy access to the drug
and the seductive influence of repeated demonstration of the drug's
happy therapeutic effects."[6]

Pearson recognized the need for prevention, although he provided
no specifics. He suggested withdrawing from practice, sometimes permanently, as an alternative superior to practicing with an addiction.
He also urged health care professionals to respect the addicted person
as one who "has as much right to his health as has the victim of
venereal disease."[7]

The professional nursing organization did not adopt any statement
or take any action related to the problem of substance abuse among
nurses at that time.[8] Not until much later did nursing organizations
recognize the need to address the issue effectively.

Several decades passed before the topic of nurse addiction reappeared
in the health care literature with Isbell and White's 1953 article.[9] It
was not until 1965, however, that Garb described the qualitative and
quantitative differences in addiction between the general population
and health care professionals.[10] In noting that narcotic addiction among
nurses and physicians was a more serious problem than generally recognized, he explained that members of the general population began using

drugs for "kicks" or "highs" but that health care professionals sought relief from discomfort. Addicted nonmedical persons were most often addicted to heroin, but Demerol® was preferred by physicians and nurses. In fact, Demerol® addiction has been called the "doctors' and nurses' addiction," according to Garb.[11]

In 1966, Bloomquist and Blanchard warned physicians about the problem of addiction among nurses.[12] The authors' opening comment reflects the punitive, judgmental attitude prevalent at the time: "Most physicians find it difficult to believe that a trusted nurse could lower herself to stealing narcotics or other harmful drugs, particularly if this theft endangers her patients." However, the authors did provide some valuable information about chemically dependent health care professionals. For instance, health care professionals usually use drugs when they are alone, and they view drugs as an acceptable escape from the pressures of life. Many users also believe that because they are health care professionals, they can handle drugs without losing control. The authors went on to warn physicians that addicted nurses often substitute and dilute medications, falsify records, and forge prescriptions.

Since the 1960s, more information has emerged and progress has been made in the area of chemical dependency among nurses. In 1984, the American Nurses' Association published a report from its Task Force on Addictions and Psychological Dysfunctions.[13] The task force defined impaired practice as that which occurs when a nurse is "unable to meet the requirements of a professional code of ethics and standard of practice because cognitive, interpersonal or psychomotor skills are affected by conditions of the individual within the environment. These factors include psychiatric illness, excessive alcohol or drug use, or addiction."

Much of the literature concerning chemically dependent nurses has focused on narcotic addiction. Yet, alcohol continues to be the most widely used of all psychoactive drugs in the United States today. In their 1984 book, Bissell and Haberman asserted that alcoholism is the most common serious illness likely to affect a professional.[14]

As a result of the increasing amount of information available about chemical dependency among nurses, many nursing associations and states, through their boards of nursing and regulatory agencies, have developed programs to assist chemically dependent nurses. These programs will be discussed further in chapter 10.

Risk Factors in Nursing

Chapter 1 presented some of the risk factors within the general population for developing the disease of chemical dependency, including heredity and abnormal metabolism of alcohol. Nurses may have additional risk factors attributable to the nursing culture or to the environment in which they practice. Nurses may therefore be more vulnerable to addiction because of their environment and the risk increases if they are genetically predisposed.

The nursing culture can best be described as the accepted system of values and beliefs that nurses as a professional group hold. The process of nursing education includes not only the acquisition of a required set of practice skills and knowledge base, but also the internalization of the values and norms of the professional group. Cohen describes this process as "professional socialization."[15] He goes on to state that it is "important to recognize that professional socialization does not begin with entry into professional school, but has its roots in the earlier experiences of the person that result in the decision to join a particular occupational group."

In nursing, there is a set of ideals that produces a common set of behavioral and attitudinal attributes.[16] Some of these attitudes and behaviors can contribute to the nurse's risk of developing chemical dependency. They include the following:

- *Caregiver role:* For the nurse, the patient always comes first. Nurses are adept at taking care of others' needs, often to the exclusion of—or failure to recognize—their own. They are trained to operate on the principle that "calm is in, panic is out." This behavior is perfectly normal when the nurse is at work. Unfortunately for the nurse, it very often translates into detachment from personal feelings both on and off the job.

  Nurses often have unrealistic expectations of themselves; no matter how bad things get, they feel they must stay in control. The norm for nurses is often to work double shifts and to put themselves in situations that place them at risk. Nurses are often recognized for going above and beyond the call of duty, and such behavior is valued. Nurses learn that they are responsible for "handling" things and staying in control. These standards and expectations are often rigid, and as a result nurses learn not to share their insecurities and explore effective ways to deal with them.

- *Self-treatment:* When nurses are ill, they often treat themselves or ignore their symptoms. All too frequently they fail to seek care or an objective evaluation of their problems. This response is due in part to their care-giving "patient-first" orientation. Taking care of personal needs is not a high priority for many nurses.

- *Pharmaceutical perspective:* Nurses respect the effectiveness of drugs. Every day on the job, they see how drugs relieve pain, anxiety, and infection. Thus, many nurses believe that mood-altering drugs such as alcohol are perfectly acceptable ways to relieve stress. High stress characterizes today's health care environment, and nurses are being asked and expected to do more with less. As stress levels increase, some nurses turn to drugs for relief.

In addition to these factors, nurses have traditionally received very little education on how to recognize chemical dependency and treat it as part of patient care. Moreover, little if any attention is given to how nurses may be at risk for developing the disease. A study of nursing schools indicated that in 57 percent of the schools responding, the average time spent on chemical dependency education was five or fewer hours. "The relatively small number of required hours in substance abuse content appears to be disproportionate to the scope and prevalence of the problems present in the patient population."[17]

Prevalence of Addiction

How many nurses are chemically dependent? Some nurses are in state alternative or diversion programs, which provide monitoring and educational programs for dealing with chemically dependent nurses. However, because states are just starting to launch these programs, data-gathering efforts are just getting under way. The terms *alternative* and *diversion* refer to the fact that the programs provide alternatives to taking disciplinary action against chemically dependent nurses. Also, some nurses have been reported to state boards of nursing for disciplinary action, but state boards may not directly identify chemical dependency as the problem.

Even if accurate numbers were available from these sources, they would only represent nurses who have been identified. Due to many factors—including denial by addicted nurses that they even have a problem, enabling behaviors by friends and colleagues who "protect" them, and lack of education about the nature of chemical dependency among health care professionals—these estimates are low.

Estimates of the prevalence of chemical dependency among nurses range from 6 to 20 percent. The lifetime risk for health care professionals becoming chemically dependent is 10 to 20 percent.[18] The American Nurses' Association has estimated that 8 to 10 percent of nurses have a drug or alcohol problem.[19] That means there could be as many as 200,000 chemically dependent nurses in the United States.[20] Some addiction specialists believe that all these estimates are conservative.

Characteristics of the Chemically Dependent Nurse

Very little research has been conducted to date on chemically dependent nurses. Therefore, it is too early to develop an accurate profile of the addicted nurse. A 1988 survey, however, provided valuable information on recovering nurses.[21] The sample included 139 recovering chemically dependent nurses and 384 non-chemically dependent nurses. Participants in the study received survey questionnaires by mail and replied anonymously. Significant differences between the two groups were as follows:

- The most significant difference involved sexual trauma and related problems. Almost 30 percent more chemically dependent than non-chemically dependent nurses reported that they had been sexually abused some time in their lives. A sizable 65 percent more reported sexual dysfunctions or illnesses, out-of-wedlock pregnancies, abortions, or miscarriages.
- Many more chemically dependent nurses had a family history of chemical dependency, parents who died from the effects of substance abuse or by suicide, and mothers who suffered from depression.
- Fifteen percent more chemically dependent nurses were "not surprised so many nurses burned out."
- Eleven percent more chemically dependent nurses were homosexuals.
- Ten percent more chemically dependent nurses were male.
- Many chemically dependent nurses had sought psychiatric help for depression, suicide attempts, emotional problems, and family crises at some time in their lives. None felt that psychotherapy helped them before they started receiving treatment for chemical dependency.

There were also important similarities:

- Ninety percent of both groups ranked nursing as highly or fairly stressful.
- Both groups agreed on the causes of stress among nurses:
  - Excessive workload
  - Proximity to illness and death
  - Difficult relationships with supervisors and physicians
- Thirty percent of both groups of respondents indicated that they had graduated in the top 10 percent of their nursing school classes.
- Ten percent of both groups had master's or doctoral degrees.

Additional survey findings show how recovering nurses viewed their disease and how they typically obtained drugs:

- Most chemically dependent nurses started using alcohol or other drugs to help them relax or reduce pain, not for recreation or in response to peer pressure.
- Symptoms of the disease reported by 75 percent of chemically dependent nurses included the following:
  - Preoccupation with alcohol or other drugs
  - Reduced attention on the job
  - Irritability
  - Frequent absenteeism or tardiness
- They reported that they obtained drugs from the following sources:
  - Patients' supplies
  - Hospital's supplies
  - Legal prescriptions
  - Forged prescriptions
  - Friends

Sullivan's findings illustrate the multidimensional nature of chemical dependency. The educational similarities between both groups also contradict the general stereotype of an alcoholic or addict as uneducated. In addition, Sullivan's study reinforces other research showing that nurses start taking drugs and alcohol for different reasons than does the general population.

Further research like Sullivan's should contribute to the development of a profile of the chemically dependent nurse. Profiles, in turn, may help nurse managers identify chemically dependent staff members earlier.

The Cost of Addiction

Chemical dependency exacts a high cost in both human and economic terms. The chemically dependent nurse and those around him pay for that dependency. Although the economic costs of addiction can be measured more easily, the human cost to the nurse and to patients, family, friends, and co-workers is substantial. The human toll includes increased stress, low morale, shame, physical and psychological diseases and complications, family dysfunction and disintegration, low self-esteem, job loss, accidents, and suicide. In fact, a California study found that from 1979 through 1981 the leading cause of death among nurses was suicide.[22]

LaGodna and Hendrix analyzed the economic cost of impaired nursing practice to the employer, the individual nurse, and the profession.[23] According to their study, impaired practice could result from substance abuse or psychological dysfunction. In arriving at their cost figures, the researchers considered all the activities and resources required when a nurse's practice is impaired and formulated the following estimates:

Employer	$17,867
Individual nurse	31,953
Board of nursing	4,300
Total:	$54,120

Researchers found that the economic cost to the employer was greatest when impaired practice, regardless of cause, went unrecognized and resulted in crises that demanded intervention.

LaGodna and Hendrix concluded that impaired nursing practice affects "turnover and retention rates, benefits, staff morale, and high level management time, as well as the quality of patient care." They added, "Prevention and early intervention strategies that could reduce or eliminate many of these costs are beginning to be defined, but their implementation is rare."[24]

At a time when the health care industry is experiencing critical problems, including decreasing financial resources and a shortage of nurses, effective solutions to nurse addiction must be applied that will benefit the employer, the nurse, and the profession. Early identification and treatment of chemically dependent nurses, retention of recovering nurses, and management of risk factors in the work environment offer the greatest promise.

Summary

Chemical dependency among nurses is nothing new. Awareness of the special vulnerability of nurses to substance abuse began as early as 1906. Early articles on the subject were often written by physicians, who served as nursing educators at the time. Not until the past 10 or 20 years, however, did the literature on the subject emphasize the significant impact that chemical dependency can have on nursing practice.

Even early articles, however, noted that nurses were at risk for becoming addicted because they worked closely with addictive drugs, including morphine and cocaine. In fact, nurses' respect for the effectiveness of drugs is a major risk factor in their developing chemical dependency. Other risk factors, many of which are embedded in the nursing culture, include these:

- The belief that the patient always comes first. This forces nurses to ignore or minimize their own problems and look for "quick fixes."
- The tendency to self-treat instead of seeking professional care. Taking care of personal needs is not a high priority among nurses; so they treat their own medical problems, with potentially harmful results.

Their lack of education on chemical dependency also puts nurses at risk. If nurses received appropriate training on the subject in nursing school, they might more readily recognize the dangers of self-medication.

Research into the general characteristics of the chemically dependent nurse is just beginning. A 1988 study of recovering nurses noted several differences between them and nurses who were not addicted. Both groups, however, rate their jobs as equally stressful. This one study pinpointed the multidimensional nature of chemical dependency and, together with future studies, may lead to the development of a comprehensive profile of the chemically dependent nurse.

The realization that impaired nursing practice entails a high economic cost was documented only recently. In a 1989 study, researchers determined that just one nurse's impaired practice could cost more than $54,000. They maintained that preventive measures and early intervention could cut costs significantly.

☐ *References*

1. Ritter, J. K. Recognition of substance abuse as a problem confronting the nursing profession. Unpublished manuscript, 1987.
2. Hyson, H. P. The moral and legal responsibilities of nurses in the purchase and prescribing of medicine. *American Journal of Nursing* 6:290–96, 1906.
3. Hyson, p. 295.
4. Ritter.
5. Pearson, C. V. How does the nurse acquire the morphine habit and how can she best obtain permanent freedom? *Trained Nurse and Hospital Review* 55:155–58, 1915.
6. Pearson, p. 155.
7. Pearson, p. 155.
8. Ritter.
9. Isbell, H., and White, W. Clinical characteristics of addiction. *American Journal of Medicine* 24:558–65, 1953.

10. Garb, S. Narcotic addiction in nurses and doctors. *Nursing Outlook* 13:30–34, Nov. 1965.

11. Garb, p. 30.

12. Bloomquist, E. R., and Blanchard, B. H. Drug abuse in the nursing profession. *GP* 34:133–39, Nov. 1966.

13. American Nurses' Association. *Addictions and Psychological Dysfunctions in Nursing.* Kansas City, MO: ANA, 1984.

14. Bissell, L., and Haberman, P. *Alcoholism in the Professions.* New York City: Oxford University Press, 1984.

15. Cohen, H. A. *The Nurse's Quest for a Professional Identity.* Reading, MA: Addison-Wesley Publishing, 1981, pp. 14–15.

16. Solari-Twadell, A. Nurse impairment: the significance of the professional culture. *Quality Review Bulletin* 14(4):103–4, Apr. 1988.

17. Heineman, E. M., and Hoffman, A. L. Substance abuse in schools of nursing: a national survey. Research presented at the Emory University Annual Conference on the Impaired Nurse, Atlanta, Mar. 1986.

18. Canfield, T. Drug addiction of health professionals. *Journal of the Association of Operating Room Nurses* 24:665–71, Oct. 1976.

19. ANA.

20. Morse, R. M., Martin, M. A., Swenson, W. M., and Niven, R. G. Prognosis of physicians treated for alcoholism or drug dependencies. *Journal of the American Medical Association* 251(6):743–46, June 1984.

21. Sullivan, E. A descriptive study of nurses recovering from chemical dependency. *Archives of Psychiatric Nursing* 1(3):194–200, June 1987.

22. Kizer, K. W., Kelter, A., Lera, G., Mitchell, D. W., and Doebbert, G. California Bureau of Vital Statistics. Female mortality by occupation, 1979–81. *California Occupational Mortality,* pp. 83–84, 170–71, 1987.

23. LaGodna, G. E., and Hendrix, M. J. Impaired nurses: a cost analysis. *Journal of Nursing Administration* 19(9):13–18, Sept. 1989.

24. LaGodna and Hendrix, p. 17.

Signs and Symptoms of Chemical Dependency

Identifying the chemically dependent nurse is rarely easy, but identification is crucial if nurse managers are to help nurses who experience problems due to alcohol or other drug use. This chapter gives nurse managers the background they need to recognize nurses who may be chemically dependent. It describes various signs and symptoms of the disease, how they may be manifested in the nurse, and methods that nurses commonly use to obtain controlled drugs in the workplace. Also included are examples that illustrate the various signs and symptoms, as well as a symptoms checklist, to make identification easier.

The nurse manager who confronts a chemically dependent nurse only after seeing obvious signs of alcohol or other drug use has waited too long. Obvious signs — such as catching a nurse in the act of diverting (or stealing) controlled drugs or observing a nurse who is overtly under the influence of alcohol or drugs — usually indicate that the disease is in an advanced stage. Chemical dependency is a progressive disease. By learning to recognize its signs and symptoms and intervening as early as possible, nurse managers increase the odds that the nurse will recover successfully.

Nurse managers are only responsible for identifying inappropriate behaviors and signs of impaired practice, not for diagnosing chemical dependency or other psychological or psychiatric conditions. Diagnosis should be left to psychiatrists and other specialists who treat addiction. To supplement the information presented in this chapter on how to identify the signs and symptoms of chemical dependency, chapter 5 discusses procedures for documenting observed signs and symptoms. Chapters 6 and 7 explain methods for intervening after the manager has observed and documented symptoms.

Faulty Memory

Instances of faulty memory can be an early sign of chemical dependency. Blackouts, repression, and euphoric recall all contribute to memory problems and literally prevent nurses from remembering what happened when they were under the influence of mood-altering substances. As a result, it is virtually impossible for chemically dependent nurses to realize on their own that they have a disease, let alone that they need to seek treatment—which is why they suffer from self-delusion.

Faulty memory can be identified by an astute nurse manager. When memory problems first occur, it may be difficult to attribute them to addiction. As they recur, however, nurse managers have good reason to suspect addiction.

Blackouts

Blackouts can best be described as chemically induced periods of amnesia. They should not be confused with passing out, which is a total loss of consciousness that sometimes occurs as a result of excessive alcohol or other drug use. During a blackout, the nurse's outward behavior may appear normal, and observers often assume that he is in control. Only later does it become obvious that the nurse is unable to recall anything about the blackout period—and never will be able to.

Blackouts may occur at any time—while the nurse is assisting with medical procedures, caring for patients, traveling, or carrying out activities of daily living. No direct correlation has been found between the quantity of mood-altering substance consumed and the frequency and duration of blackouts. Blackouts may last for seconds, minutes, hours, days, or weeks.

Unpredictability is characteristic of people who are experiencing blackouts. Chemically dependent nurses become increasingly anxious, confused, afraid, and depressed as their memory losses continue. As the disease progresses, memory losses occur more frequently and unpredictably. Chemically dependent nurses anxiously ask themselves, "What did I do after I left the party?" "Where did I go to put 200 miles on my car?" Or "Why is everyone avoiding me?" They refuse to believe witnesses who tell them what they actually did during a blackout and dismiss such accounts as exaggerations or overreactions. Nevertheless their anxiety level increases.

After several blackouts, chemically dependent nurses begin to fear that they are going crazy, and so they force themselves to black out the blackouts. Their delusional system is so effective that they believe everyone draws a blank whenever they have had too much to drink. However, the truth is that "the willingness to tolerate repeated black-outs as a normal part of life rarely if ever occurs in the absence of chemical dependency."[1]

For example, one recovering nurse described a blackout he had experienced years earlier this way. He had a long history of alcohol and Demerol® use. His last memory was that he began taking Demerol® on Thursday night while he was working as a nursing supervisor at a local hospital. When he "came to" he was on an airplane. He did not know what day it was, where he was going, how he got on the plane, or anything else. He felt confused, anxious, and scared. He had no idea whether he was going to some unknown place or coming home. Too embarrassed and ashamed to ask the flight attendant for help, he checked his pockets for clues instead. His plane ticket indicated a round-trip fare from Nashville to New York. He also found an American Express receipt for $580 in purchases from Bloomingdale's and a receipt from a New York City hotel.

Armed only with this information, he was able to conclude that it was Sunday. Putting all the clues together, he figured out that he had left Nashville on Thursday, spent three days in New York City, shopped at Bloomingdale's, and was finally on his way home. Even with the receipts as reminders, he had no recollection of when he decided to go to New York, how he got to the airport, how he spent those three days, where he went, what he did, whether he had a good time, or anything else. And he got no consolation when he went to the baggage claim area, where he found no packages from Bloomingdale's and no sympathy from the baggage handlers.

Not every nurse who blacks out ends up going so far or losing so much time. Blackouts may involve conversations, nursing procedures, phone calls, meetings, and assignments. They may last minutes or days. The danger to chemically dependent nurses and the patients under their care is all too obvious.

Repression

In the context of chemical dependency, *repression* can be defined as a psychologically induced period of amnesia. It differs from blackouts, which are chemically induced. However, the end result is the same — a loss of memory.

For example, a nurse may feel so much guilt and shame after physically abusing her child while under the influence of drugs that she represses her feelings as well as her conscious recollection of the beatings. The pain generated by these emotions is so great that the nurse is unable to face it, and so she represses every memory of these episodes. Repression actually becomes a survival skill.

The feelings that nurses seek to repress are brought on by their addiction. They do not acknowledge the addiction or the fact that they have a disease. All they know is that they are doing things that cause painful emotions, including shame, guilt, and remorse.

Repression is not unique to chemically dependent people. Even normal people would be emotionally overwhelmed if they remembered all the shameful and embarrassing events in their lives. Often, the normal repression of embarrassing or shameful memories is of little consequence because the behavior is not repeated. With addicted nurses, however, the behavior keeps repeating itself and so does the repression, which usually manifests itself in observable signs of nervousness, resentment, self-destructive tendencies, self-pity, or suicidal tendencies.[2]

Euphoric Recall

Euphoria can be defined as a feeling of heightened well-being or elation. As their disease progresses, chemically dependent nurses often recall drinking or drug-using episodes euphorically. Although they believe that they remember everything that happened, actually all they remember is how they felt, which is generally pleasant. They have no memory of their slurred speech, stumbling gait, or hostility, and they trust that their recollections are accurate.

Euphoric recall, therefore, makes it impossible for addicted nurses to accurately judge their abilities under the influence of mood-altering chemicals. They simply are not aware that they cannot do everything that they are capable of doing when not under the influence of drugs. Later, they believe that they acted or performed as usual.

For example, Martha, an emergency department nurse, had been drinking heavily for three years. During that time, she had progressed from "stress relief" drinking to alcoholic drinking. For the past year, she had consistently come to work under the influence and often drank while on duty.

At seven one evening, three victims of an automobile accident arrived at the hospital. Martha's assignment was to start intravenous lines on the patients and monitor vital signs. When it took her three tries to start the line on the first patient, her team members became aware that something was wrong.

The nurse manager, who was floating among the three patients, noticed the obvious signs of intoxication in Martha and suggested that she take a break. Martha refused, saying that she was needed there and that she had just taken her break an hour earlier. She insisted that she was okay to work. Carole, the nurse manager, ordered Martha to leave the bedside because she was unable to provide the required care. Martha became indignant and stormed out of the department and the hospital.

When Martha arrived the next day for her regular shift, Carole called her into her office and recounted the incidents of the previous day, but Martha refused to believe what Carole told her. When Carole added that the other team members had also witnessed her intoxication, Martha vehemently denied that she had been drunk while on duty and maintained that she had been fully capable of performing her job.

People who interact with chemically dependent nurses like Martha generally assume that the nurses are aware of what is happening around them and what reality is. However, the nurses' advancing delusional state makes it virtually impossible for them to recognize the truth and seek help. It is a lifesaving gesture for those around chemically dependent nurses to intervene and break through the wall of delusion.

Denial

Perhaps the most striking and characteristic symptom of chemical dependency is denial. *Denial* in the psychological sense can be defined as an unconscious defense mechanism that allows a person to avoid the full realization of an emotionally painful fact by denying that it is true. Denial occurs outside the person's awareness, whereas lying is an intentional (conscious) distortion of the truth. For example, addicted nurses will deny that their consumption of alcohol or drugs is causing problems for them and those around them even when a nurse manager presents evidence to the contrary. They simply cannot see the consequences of their addiction.

For the chemically dependent nurse, denial is most likely to occur when reality becomes too threatening to endure. Mental health researchers do not understand all the factors that bring about denial, but one factor appears to be the nurse's inability to accept her loss of control over the use of alcohol and other drugs.[3]

Denial can be manifested in a number of ways, including minimization, rationalization, projection, and intellectualization. Nurses *minimize* their drinking or other drug use to make it seem less severe than it actually is. They might say, "I don't drink very often, only when I'm uptight after work." They would not admit that they need three drinks just to wind down after work or that it has become necessary to drink larger quantities of alcohol and to drink more frequently. Or they might say, "Cocaine isn't a problem for me. I'm just a recreational user." They would not mention that it is costing them more and more of their salary every week and presenting problems at home.

When nurses who are chemically dependent become uncomfortable with their drug or alcohol use, they may *rationalize* it in an effort to make it seem more acceptable. For example, a nurse might say, "If you had to deal with the stress I have on my job, you'd drink, too," when for the past year, he had been drinking beer as soon as he got home from work. What started as one or two beers with friends a few times a week had progressed to drinking beer alone at home until he passed out.

Projection occurs when the nurse denies responsibility for her own chemical abuse by putting—or projecting—the blame onto other people. That is, whatever is unacceptable is attributed to someone else. For example, a chemically dependent nurse might say, "Why are you picking on me? I'm not the one with the problem. You are."

Chemically dependent nurses frequently use *intellectualization* to make the unreasonable seem reasonable by explaining it away. For instance, they might say something like "I only have a couple of drinks before I come in to work. It helps me to relax and deal with the stress on the unit much better. I am able to respond to situations more effectively. I couldn't work as well without it and so it makes perfect sense to me."

Many people use defense mechanisms such as these when they experience anxiety and fear or feel threatened. Used occasionally, defense mechanisms can reduce our natural anxiety and fear, enable us to get through difficult situations, and allow us to continue to function normally. When defense mechanisms are used continually to cope with everyday life, however, they can alter our perceptions of reality. This often is the case with chemically dependent people.

These four methods of denial block chemically dependent nurses' awareness of their disease. By keeping them out of touch with reality, denial makes it impossible for them to understand that they have a problem and, most often, unlikely for them to seek help.

Growing Preoccupation with Drugs

As a chemically dependent nurse's disease progresses, her relationship with her drug of choice changes. What may have started as social or medical use becomes a growing preoccupation. For example, the dosage of drug available through her physician's prescription is no longer effective or the prescription has expired. She turns to self-medication by diverting hospital supplies or getting staff physicians to write additional prescriptions. The nurse's goal at this stage of chemical dependency is to obtain the drugs she needs; no longer is it a matter of choice.

Usage patterns also change. For example, instead of waiting until after work to do their heavy drinking, alcoholic nurses may drink during their lunch hours or breaks. Addicts lose control over their drug use or drinking and use as often as possible, even on the job.

As using alcohol or other drugs becomes the most important aspect of their lives, chemically dependent nurses begin structuring their lives around their addictions. They avoid places, situations, and assignments that preclude use of alcohol or drugs and seek out those where such use will be easy, that is, where controls on controlled drugs are lax. Nurses whose source of drugs is the hospital often choose to work on units where controlled drugs are readily available (surgery, intensive care, coronary care, and orthopedics, for example).

The need for a ready supply of drugs often leads addicted nurses to hoard, hide, or ration their supplies. Nurses whose drug of choice is alcohol often hide bottles in their purses, bags, or lockers. Common drugs or preparations that contain alcohol, such as cough syrup and mouthwash, should not be overlooked as a source of supply. Nurses who are dependent on narcotics or pharmaceutical drugs have instant access to them on practically every patient unit.

For example, a nurse with a nine-month history of narcotic addiction diverted an average of 800 milligrams of Demerol® during her day shift on a busy medical center intensive care unit. She claimed that she never used drugs while on duty, but still a great deal of her workday was spent figuring out how to get the Demerol® without being detected and then actually obtaining it. As soon as she arrived home, she injected 300 milligrams, using the remaining supply over the course of the evening. She consistently reported to work on her assigned shifts and felt that her practice was not affected by her drug use.

Even though the nurse did not use Demerol® while she was on duty, a great deal of time and attention was given to self-medication while at work to overcome the effects of withdrawal, and she was continually preoccupied during work hours with diverting drugs undetected. The time spent on drug-related concerns was time spent away from delivering good patient care. Much of the care she did deliver was compromised by her divided concentration. Impaired practice is a real threat whenever anything less than high-quality care is given and whenever the nurse's attention is focused on concerns other than patient care.

Isolation

Isolation becomes more and more apparent as chemical dependency advances. Chemically dependent nurses feel very alone, even in a crowd.

In fact, drug use is seldom a social event, especially when the drugs were diverted from the workplace. With the exception of early alcohol use, nurses usually drink or use drugs alone and withdraw from contact with peers. They avoid lunches or breaks with co-workers and do not socialize with co-workers outside of work.

Tolerance

As their addiction worsens, nurses develop a growing physical tolerance for alcohol or other drugs. To achieve the desired high, or mood change, they must increase the amount of alcohol or other substance consumed. All too often, people erroneously believe that someone able to consume large amounts of alcohol or other drugs without appearing to be high does not have a problem. Actually, it takes an even greater quantity of chemicals to produce the sought-after, mood-altering effect.

Rapid and Spontaneous Use

Another symptom of dependency is rapid and spontaneous use. Chemically dependent nurses, for whom getting the drug becomes an overpowering and all-consuming need, start looking for quick results. Many use drugs impulsively and often at great risk.

Consider the nurse on duty who diverts Demerol® at the change of shifts or substitutes Phenergan® for Demerol® for postoperative patients and then goes to the restroom and injects the Demerol® while still on duty. This behavior is an obvious indication that the disease has taken control. Ultimately, no risk is too great if the result is getting the drugs that are so desperately needed.

Deterioration in Several Areas of Life

As the disease of chemical dependency progresses, relationships and work performance often deteriorate. Relationships with family, friends, supervisors, and co-workers change. Chemically dependent nurses tend to withdraw from social, family, and work-related activities. Increases in the incidence of divorce, family dysfunction, and child rebellion are common. The effects of the disease on those around the chemically dependent nurse can be as profound as the effects on the nurse himself.

Usually, the nurse experiences family and personal problems before the alcohol or other drug use becomes apparent in the workplace. Nurse managers who are aware of the following problems in a nurse's private life might be warranted in suspecting chemical abuse:

- Spouse or child abuse
- Driving under the influence (DUI) of alcohol or drugs
- Family history of chemical dependency
- Decreased socialization with friends and increased isolation
- Frequent automobile accidents
- Frequent accidents, injuries, and illnesses
- Legal problems

Deteriorating job performance may also be a sign of chemical dependency. Even though the nurse may appear to be doing satisfactory work, in many cases, he may be increasingly unreliable and unpredictable. Chemical dependency affects an individual's job performance in four areas that are the key aspects of every nurse's practice:

- Work-related knowledge and memory retrieval
- Physical abilities
- Communication skills
- Observation skills

Specific signs that may indicate deteriorating job performance related to chemical dependency include the following:

- Missed deadlines and difficulty meeting schedules
- Inattention to standards of care
- Neglected details, increased number of errors, and poor judgment
- Co-workers' complaints about poor performance, inappropriate behavior, or alcohol or other drug use
- Increased number of breaks
- Disorganized, unsteady, or erratic work pace
- Refusal or reluctance to work overtime among alcoholic nurses
- Eagerness to work overtime or tendency to arrive early, leave late, or skip lunch among drug-dependent nurses
- Blaming of co-workers for poor performance
- Difficulty following instructions
- Difficulty concentrating as manifested by:
  - Needing to exert greater effort to accomplish the usual amount of work
  - Taking more time to complete tasks
  - Making repeated mistakes due to inattention
  - Forgetting important information
- Less work accomplished with less enthusiasm
- Increased difficulty in handling complex assignments
- Difficulty following instructions, details, and conversations

37

- Job assignments refused or left incomplete
- Improbable excuses for poor job performance
- Complaints from patients and families, such as:
  - Poor or reduced relief from analgesics
  - Lack of attention or poor care from a particular nurse
  - Rude or inappropriate behavior on the part of a particular nurse
  - Discrepancies between patient's and nurse's reports concerning administration of medications
- Decreased quality of nurse's notes as evidenced by:
  - Numerous errors
  - Poor handwriting
  - Discrepancies between written and oral reports
  - Illogical comments and notations
  - Blatant omissions
- Avoidance of co-workers and supervisors
- Money borrowed from co-workers

Physical Symptoms

Nurses who suffer from chemical dependency also may exhibit a wide range of physical symptoms. Some are readily observable, but others can be detected only through medical evaluation. It is important to remember that some chemically dependent nurses may not exhibit serious physical symptoms even in the later stages of the disease. The following physical symptoms and medical problems may be signs of chemical dependency:

- Nausea, vomiting, and diarrhea
- Slurred speech
- Tremors
- Anxiety and spaciness
- Chronic hangover
- Odor of alcohol on breath
- Diaphoresis and flushed face
- Sniffling, sneezing, and watery eyes
- Unusual, unexplained weight loss or gain
- Frequent complaints of illness or pain
- Excessive bruises on arms, ankles, and hands
- Frequent hospitalizations
- Repeated minor injuries on and off the job
- Higher-than-average accident rate

Behavioral Changes

The following behavioral changes may also indicate addiction:

- Wide mood swings, depression, and threatened or attempted suicide
- Sleeping on the job
- Difficulty conceptualizing
- Staggering gait
- Inattention to personal appearance
- Increased irritability
- Reduced eye contact
- Elaborate rationalizations
- Unreasonable resentments
- Controlling behaviors and inflexibility
- Lies, defensiveness, and suspiciousness
- Overreaction to criticism
- Unreliability
- Frequent conflicts with supervisor and co-workers
- Isolation from friends and co-workers and eating alone
- Frequent use of breath mints and mouthwashes
- Alternate periods of high and low productivity
- Frequent trips to restroom and unexplained absences
- Attendance problems (typical of the alcoholic nurse or the nurse whose drug of choice is not obtained from the workplace):
  - Prolonged and/or unpredictable absences from the work area
  - Excessive lateness
  - Long lunches and breaks
  - Early departures
  - Frequent absences before and after weekends and holidays
  - Frequent absences for vague or improbable reasons
- Unusual attendance behaviors (typical of nurses who obtain their drug supply at work):
  - Disappearances from the unit
  - Appearances on the unit on days off

Very often, changes in the nurse's behavior and job performance are so subtle and gradual that managers may overlook them or attribute them to personal problems. Nurse managers should ask themselves, "Is this normal or acceptable behavior for a nurse in this situation?" Any deviation from acceptable procedures and behaviors should serve as a red flag to indicate possible problems. A red flag may not always indicate chemical dependency, but it usually does mean that something is wrong. It should at least alert managers to the need to observe the nurse more closely until the puzzle pieces fit together.

The Workplace as a Source of Supply

The health care workplace is often the source of supply for chemically dependent nurses. They have access to pharmaceutical drugs on the patient unit or in the pharmacy drug supply. Alcohol and drugs may also be obtained from other hospital employees. Furthermore, because health care facilities are usually busy places, people other than staff and visitors may enter the facility and carry on drug dealing undetected. This possibility should not be overlooked.

Alcohol

Alcohol is available in the health care workplace in preparations such as cough syrup and mouthwash. The alcoholic nurse's pattern of use frequently includes drinking before reporting for duty and continuing to ingest alcohol during breaks and meals as needed. A supply of alcohol may be brought to the workplace and kept in a purse, bag, or locker. It also may be mixed with acceptable beverages such as coffee and soda and consumed openly in the hospital. Most often, the nurse chooses alcohol that she believes to be undetectable on her breath—for example, vodka. Even those alcoholic nurses who do not drink immediately before coming to work or during work hours have problems resulting from chronic alcohol withdrawal and hangovers that affect their job performance and safe practice.

Undiverted Prescription Drugs

Chemically dependent nurses can obtain prescription drugs in the workplace without diverting them from the patients' supplies or the unit's controlled drug cabinet. This can be done in the following ways:

- *They obtain prescriptions from staff physicians.* A nurse may approach a doctor on the unit and say, "I'm having problems with my back today, what with all this patient lifting. Could you give me a little Valium®?" Unaware of the nurse's real problem and reluctant to say no, the physician writes out a prescription. The physician may rationalize this act by thinking, "He's a professional colleague and knows what he needs. There won't be any problems."

- *They obtain prescriptions from emergency department physicians,* who very often handle employee health needs. The nurse may claim to have had an accident and go to the physician for help. Or she may simply ask for relief from a somatic complaint.
- *They steal patients' medications.* Patients admitted to the hospital often bring their own supplies of prescription medications. Hospital policy usually dictates that the medications be turned over to a nurse and locked in the unit's drug cabinet until the patient is discharged. The admitting nurse or any other nurse with access to the drug cabinet can easily take the drugs for her own use. By the time the patient is discharged, it is usually difficult to track the missing medications. The emergency department is often the easiest place to take patients' medications without detection.
- *They forge prescriptions.* Chemically dependent nurses (or nurses obtaining drugs for others) may call prescriptions in to private pharmacies and obtain prescription drugs.

Forging prescriptions is relatively easy. For example, a nurse working in the admissions office of a nursing home routinely called prescriptions in to a local pharmacy for the residents. As an employee, she could also receive her own prescriptions at reduced cost.

For six months, the nurse called in a Valium® prescription for herself without a physician's order and used her own name. Because of the numerous charges to her account, however, she eventually became concerned that she might get caught. So on one occasion she called in her prescription using another nurse's name.

Within a few weeks, the nurse in whose name the Valium® was ordered questioned the charge to her personal account, and through an internal investigation, the chemically dependent nurse's prescription forgery was discovered. The nursing home also discovered her two-year history of Valium® dependency. Within days, she was in treatment.

Diverted Prescription Drugs

Drugs prescribed for patients while they are in a health care facility can be diverted, or stolen, in a number of ways, including:

- Directly from patients by:
  - Replacing medications with substitutes such as Phenergan®, Vistaril®, and saline
  - Giving patients partial doses combined with Phenergan® or saline

- From the unit's drug supply by:
  - Substituting saline or other substances for controlled drugs in multiple-dose vials or unit doses
  - Signing out controlled drugs for patients for whom there is no physician's order
  - Signing out controlled drugs for discharged or transferred patients
  - Signing out controlled drugs and backdating records
  - Altering physicians' orders
  - Writing verbal orders without a physician's authorization
  - Signing out prn ("as needed") controlled drugs for patients who have not requested them
  - Signing out prn controlled drugs for patients who then refuse the medication
  - Stealing discarded unit dose syringes
  - Stealing the unit's controlled drug allotment
  - Stealing drugs during shift changes
  - Stealing drugs from surgical areas
  - Theft from unsecured narcotics storage areas
  - Theft of noncontrolled mood-altering drugs
- From the pharmacy by using presigned prescription forms that are locked in the narcotics box

The following signs may indicate that drug diversion is taking place:

- Errors in controlled drug count
- Apparent tampering with controlled drug vials
- Unwitnessed or excessive drug waste, loss, or breakage
- Increased complaints of ineffective pain control from patients
- Signature variations on controlled drug records (forgeries)
- Increased quantity of drugs required on unit
- Discrepancies among physicians' orders, progress notes, and controlled drug records
- Above-average number of signouts on controlled drug sheets
- Numerous corrections in controlled drug records
- Higher patient prn doses than on other shifts
- Controlled drugs given to patients on day of discharge when they had not requested them on previous days/shifts
- Medications signed out for patients discharged or transferred to another unit

In addition, chemically dependent nurses may give medication to patients assigned to other nurses without being requested to do so, or they may behave defensively when questioned about medications they administered.

Patterns of Symptoms

No single sign or symptom necessarily indicates chemical dependency in a nurse, but a combination of several signs or symptoms may. The checklist in figure 3-1 (pp. 44–45) can be used to identify a pattern in the signs and symptoms that nurse managers and co-workers have noticed in a particular nurse.

Figure 3-2 (pp. 46–47) groups signs and symptoms into patterns according to the stages of alcoholism. The stages illustrated in the figure reflect the behavioral patterns of the heavy drinker and the dependent drinker and show the progressing problems described in Johnson's stage three, harmful dependency, and stage four, alcohol use to feel normal (refer to chapter 1). Note that the job efficiency percentages in figure 3-2 demonstrate a marked decline in the later stages of the disease.

Keep in mind that many of the signs on the checklist in figure 3-1 can indicate personal or emotional problems as well as chemical dependency. Using the checklist and comparing the results to figure 3-2 does not provide a diagnosis of chemical dependency. As mentioned earlier, a nurse manager is not responsible for diagnosing a nurse's problem but for intervening in order to resolve the problem. Therefore, if the symptoms resemble those described in this chapter, the manager should intervene and explain to the nurse that "according to hospital policy, the first thing we do in cases like this is rule out alcohol or other drug dependencies." If the addictions specialist who examines the nurse reports that chemical dependency is not the problem, the nurse manager can then explore other referral options, for example, for psychiatric or psychological care. (See chapter 7 for an in-depth discussion of the process of intervention.)

Summary

Because chemically dependent nurses are most often in denial and unable to ask for help, nurse managers must do so on their behalf. Once managers do, they can effectively prepare to intervene and interrupt the progression of a devastating but treatable disease. By being aware of the signs and symptoms outlined in this chapter, the nurse manager has a better chance of intervening during the early stages of the disease, when the potential for a successful recovery is the greatest.

Figure 3-1. Checklist of Unsatisfactory Nursing Performance

Review the list below. Place a check mark next to each situation that pertains to the nurse about whom you are concerned.

I. Absenteeism

_____ Instances of leaving without permission
_____ Excessive sick leave
_____ Frequent Monday and/or Friday absences
_____ Repeated absences, particularly when they follow a pattern
_____ Lateness to work, especially on Monday mornings, and/or returning from lunch
_____ Leaving work early
_____ Peculiar and increasingly unbelievable excuses for absences or lateness
_____ Absent more often than other employees for colds, flu, gastritis, and so forth
_____ Frequent unscheduled short-term absences (with or without medical explanation)

II. "On-the-Job" Absenteeism

_____ Continued absences from post more than job requires—"goofing off"
_____ Long coffee breaks, lunch breaks
_____ Repeated undealt-with physical illness on the job
_____ Frequent trips to the restroom

III. Uneven Work Pattern

_____ Alternate periods of high and low productivity

IV. High Accident Rate

_____ Accidents on the job
_____ Accidents off the job (but affecting job performance)
_____ "Horseplay" that causes unsafe conditions

V. Problems with Memory

_____ Difficulty in recalling instructions, details, conversations, and so forth
_____ Difficulty recalling nurse's own mistakes

VI. Difficulty in Concentration

_____ Work requiring greater effort
_____ Jobs taking more time
_____ Repeated mistakes due to inattention
_____ Bad decisions or poor judgment
_____ Errors in charting
_____ Forgetfulness

VII. Confusion

_____ Difficulty following instructions
_____ Increasing difficulty handling complex assignments

Figure 3-1. (Continued)

VIII. Reporting to Work in an Inappropriate State

_____ Coming to/returning to work in an obviously altered condition

IX. General Lowered Job Efficiency

_____ Missed deadlines, unreliability
_____ Complaints from patients, family members
_____ Improbable excuses for poor job performance
_____ Undependability
_____ Refusal to take job assignments, failure to complete assignments

X. Poor Employee Relationships on the Job

_____ Failure to keep promises; unreasonable excuses for failing to keep promises
_____ Overreaction to real or imagined criticism
_____ Borrowing money from co-workers
_____ Unreasonable resentments
_____ Avoidance of associates
_____ Lying and exaggerating
_____ Complaints from co-workers, supervisors, other staff
_____ Blaming others for problems

XI. Inappropriate Appearance

_____ Decreased attention to personal appearance and hygiene
_____ Odor of alcohol on breath
_____ Glassy, red eyes
_____ Tremors

XII. Other Problem Behaviors

_____ Sleeping on the job
_____ Withdrawal from others, self-isolation
_____ Mood swings
_____ Increasing irritability
_____ Problems at home, with relationships, with finances

XIII. Drug Diversion

_____ Consistent volunteering to give medications
_____ Patient complaints of no relief; discrepancies on records
_____ Consistent administration of IM (prn) and maximum doses when other nurses do not demonstrate such patterns
_____ Frequent wastage, such as spilling drugs or breaking vials
_____ Unobserved wastage, no cosignatures
_____ Work on a unit where drugs are missing or have been tampered with
_____ Frequent volunteering for additional shifts; appearing on unit when not assigned

Figure 3-2. How an Alcoholic Employee Behaves

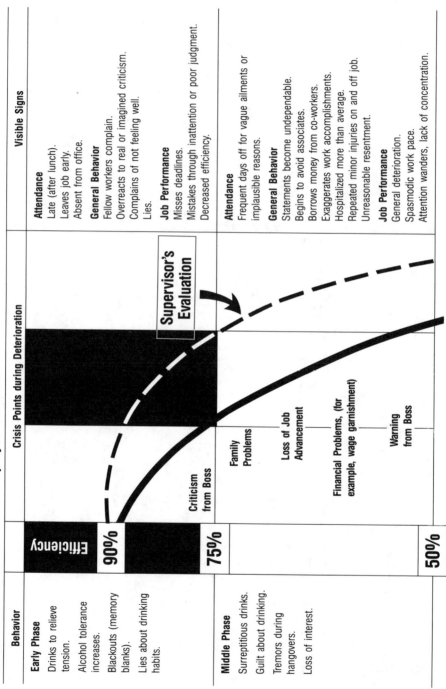

Late Middle Phase
Avoids discussion of problem.
Fails in efforts at control.
Neglects food.
Prefers to drink alone.

Late Phase
Believes that other activities interfere with his drinking.

25%

In Trouble with Law

Typical Crisis

Punitive Disciplinary Action

Serious Family Problems—Separation

Serious Financial Problems

Final Warning from Boss

Area of Greatest Coverup

Termination

Hospitalization

Attendance
Frequent time off, sometimes for several days.
Fails to return from lunch.

General Behavior
Grandiose, aggressive, or belligerent.
Domestic problems interfere with work.
Apparent loss of ethical values.
Money problems, garnishment of salary.
Hospitalization increases.
Refuses to discuss problems.
Trouble with the law.

Job Performance
Far below expected level.

Attendance
Prolonged unpredictable absences.

General Behavior
Drinking on job.
Totally undependable.
Repeated hospitalization.
Visible physical deterioration.
Money problems worse.
Serious family problems and/or divorce.

Job Performance
Uneven and generally incompetent.

Increasing dependency over time

47

☐ *References*

1. Johnson, V. *Intervention: How to Help Someone Who Doesn't Want Help.* Minneapolis: Johnson Institute, 1986.
2. Johnson.
3. Twerski, A. *It Happens to Doctors Too.* Center City, MN: Hazelden, 1982.

Enabling, an Obstacle
to Identification and Intervention

After graduating from nursing school, Dave began to practice as a full-time registered nurse in the emergency department of a large metropolitan medical center. He was well liked by his peers and held in high regard as a competent and caring nurse by co-workers, supervisors, and physicians. Unknown to his peers, Dave was an active alcoholic who had had a "drinking problem" throughout nursing school.

For a number of years, Dave hid his addiction successfully from his co-workers by being a "supernurse." As his disease progressed, however, his job performance started slipping. He began missing deadlines and frequently transcribed physicians' orders incorrectly. He was also short-tempered with both patients and staff, left incomplete and inappropriate nursing notes, and failed to follow treatment protocols. His job performance and attitude became inconsistent and unpredictable.

Dave's co-workers noticed the change in his behavior. They knew that he had some kind of problem, and most of them knew that he was a "heavy drinker." Because they cared about him and didn't want him to get into trouble, they covered for him. Fellow nurses followed behind him and checked his work, apologized to patients when he was having a "bad day," and ran interference with physicians. When the unit supervisor commented on his absenteeism, Dave's co-workers made excuses for him.

Dave's supervisor expressed increasing concern and irritation with his regular tardiness and absenteeism. As a result, the staff became concerned that Dave might lose his job, and so they decided to take turns making sure that he got to work on time.

On the days he was scheduled to work, they called him a half-hour before his shift started to make sure that he was up. Most often, the calls woke him in time to make it to work on schedule. When there was no answer, a staff member would go to Dave's house, which was across the street from the hospital, and wake him up. Frequently, Dave was found sleeping in the same clothes he had worn the day before.

Despite all his co-workers' good intentions, caring, and covering up, Dave got worse. Eventually, he was fired by the hospital's director of nursing. In her termination meeting with Dave, she told him that even though he was a good nurse and everyone cared about him, he had a serious problem that the hospital couldn't deal with. She added that if he could get himself straightened out, the hospital would be glad to rehire him.

Dave was not able to "straighten himself out." After hopping from job to job for three years, he was finally confronted by a supervisor who recognized the destructive pattern of chemical dependency. Dave then entered treatment. Four years into recovery, he returned to the first hospital from which he was fired. Since that time, he has continued to do well in recovery and consistently receives commendations for his outstanding nursing practice.

This story ends well, but Dave should have entered treatment much earlier. One reason he did not was because his co-workers "enabled," or protected, him. Their lack of knowledge and understanding about chemical dependency and the nature of the disease were the primary reasons for their enabling behavior, cover-up activities, and delayed intervention. Fortunately, enabling can stop when people understand how much it harms rather than helps the chemically dependent person.

What Is Enabling?

Chemical dependency affects not only the addicted nurse; it also deeply affects those close to her — family, co-workers, and friends. Although the chemically dependent person may withdraw from family, friends, and social situations as the disease progresses, associated problems typically affect at least 10 other people. That number may be even higher for addicted nurses because of the number of social and professional systems in which nurses are involved. (See figure 4-1.)

Family members, friends, supervisors, and co-workers become involved in the maze of problems a chemically dependent nurse experiences. As the disease progresses, the nurse's problems and behaviors become more difficult for those around him, and these same people often unwittingly contribute to that progression by their enabling behavior.

Enabling, as the term is used in the chemical dependency field, refers to any behavior, no matter how well intentioned, that shields or prevents the addict from experiencing the consequences of his alcohol or other drug use. Usually we think of enabling as a positive action

Figure 4-1. Multiple-System Interactions of the Chemically Dependent Nurse

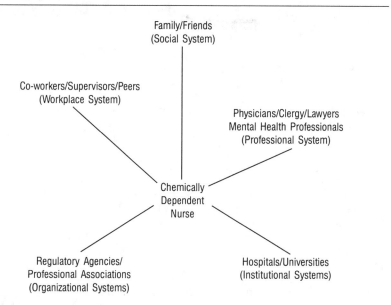

that encourages or empowers an individual to accomplish a goal. Unfortunately, for chemically dependent nurses, enabling reinforces their denial that alcohol or other drugs are a problem. The disease worsens as a result.

In fact, enabling behavior is such a powerful "aid" to chemically dependent nurses that they cannot continue abusing drugs or alcohol successfully without an enabler. Enablers defend, protect, and cover up for them. Individuals and groups, even institutions, can all be enablers. Enabling is not a deliberate, conscious process but rather a learned response. Very often enablers are repeating patterns they learned as children: to keep the peace at all costs, to put up a brave front, to keep family problems at home, and to protect those they care about from pain and suffering. For the most part, enabling behaviors seem like the natural and right thing to do. However, enablers are the primary obstacle to getting chemically dependent nurses the help that they need. No one wins or benefits from enabling—neither the chemically dependent nurse who gets worse nor the enabler who feels used, exhausted, and powerless.

How and why enabling happens is a complicated question. This chapter focuses on how to recognize it and how it affects the role of nurse managers. An effective way to begin understanding enabling and its consequences is in terms of the family, where enabling invariably takes place. The nursing unit most often functions and behaves in much the same way that a family does.

Family Members as Enablers

As the disease of chemical dependency enters increasingly debilitating stages, the level of family dysfunction becomes more destructive, not only to the nurse but also to every other member of the family.

Four Stages of Enabling

Each family is different and may respond to the disease in its own unique way. However, there are some predictable stages through which most families pass.[1]

Stage One

Family members become anxious about the use of alcohol or other drugs and the inappropriate behaviors associated with that use. Their anxiety is manifested in increased tensions, arguments, and strained relationships. Refusing to deal openly with the underlying issue, however, the family members simply deny that their problems are due to the chemical dependency of their mother, father, son, daughter, sister, or brother.

Stage Two

The whole family becomes preoccupied with one person's alcohol or other drug use. Because they do not understand the disease, they may even believe that they are in some way responsible for causing it. As a result, they attempt to control the family member's use of mood-altering substances. Family life at this stage is unmanageable; often, social events are canceled or not attended because of the addicted member's unpredictability.

Stage Three

Family members begin to assume rigid roles in relationship to the addicted person. At this time, enabling becomes very strong, and family members develop dysfunctional behaviors and coping mechanisms, manifested as particular roles. Denial of personal feelings and needs is also common at this stage.

The person closest to the chemically dependent family member, usually the spouse, assumes the role of "chief enabler." In trying to make everything okay for other family members by covering for the addicted member, the chief enabler worries, neglects himself, and shields the addicted member as well as the rest of the family from the consequences of the drinking or other drug use.

The youngest child in such families typically becomes the "family mascot" and tries to provide some relief for the family's pain by acting as the family clown. Older siblings assume other roles. These roles, which family members use to cope with problems resulting from the addicted member's behavior, become very predictable.[2]

Stage Four

At this stage, crises usually occur as the family tries to break out of a severely dysfunctional situation that seems hopeless. This is when emotional separation, divorce, suicide, or even homicide may occur. Emotional exhaustion characterizes this stage. Nevertheless, the family still protects the chemically dependent person.

Enabling Behaviors

Families enable chemically dependent members in any or all of the following ways:

- *Denying:* Denying that alcohol or other drugs are a problem or that they are the primary problem can be so entrenched that family members deny the existence of any problem at all.
- *Minimizing:* Families minimize the problems associated with alcohol or other drug use and the negative effects of addictive behaviors.
- *Rationalizing:* Families view incidents resulting from alcohol or drug use as isolated events, not as a pattern of harmful dependency. They explain away the behaviors as due to other problems or circumstances. They attempt to find out what the "real" problem is in the belief that once it is solved, the alcohol or other drug use will disappear.
- *Avoiding:* Situations or problems that might result in alcohol or drug use or inappropriate behaviors are avoided. No one talks openly about the problem. Family members withdraw from contact with the addicted person.

- *Waiting and hoping that things will change:* The family hopes that by not actively intervening with the chemically dependent family member and not making waves, things will get better on their own.
- *Protecting:* In protecting the chemically dependent member from feeling the consequences of his behavior, the family covers up and lies for the addict, carries out the addict's responsibilities, and makes excuses to friends, employers, and others.
- *Controlling:* Families try to control the substance use by controlling the availability of alcohol or other drugs and the situations in which their use occurs.
- *Obeying the "no talk" rule:* The "family secret" is kept within the family. No one discusses the problem with anyone else, not even other relatives.

Some of these behaviors, such as denial and minimizing, are the same as actual symptoms of addiction (as explained previously in chapter 3). This is more than a coincidence in that family members "suffer" the disease of chemical dependency along with the addicted member. As the nurse's disease worsens, so does the enabling behavior; that is, the two tend to move in tandem. If a family's highly developed enabling system remains intact, the disease progresses until the nurse dies or until intervention comes from outside the family. Unfortunately, the hospital's response to a nurse's chemical dependency often parallels the enabling behavior of the family.

Co-workers as Enablers

As we saw so vividly in the case history that opened this chapter, the addicted nurse's friends and peers at work may enable addictive behavior in numerous ways, among them:

- Checking the nurse's work to avoid charges of poor performance
- Making excuses for the nurse's work or behavior to patients and supervisors
- Even making sure the nurse gets to work on time after a binge or hangover

Nurse managers may also act as enablers in important ways. Often, the enabling stems from long-held beliefs and attitudes about nurses, on the one hand, and alcoholics or addicts, on the other. Exercise 4-1 (on p. 64) is designed to help managers explore these attitudes.

Enabling Manager's Beliefs

Even nurse managers who are familiar with the disease of chemical dependency and its signs and symptoms may be reluctant to confront the nurse and refer her to a treatment program. Enabling beliefs cloud their ability to see the situation as it really is. These beliefs enable not only the dependent nurse, but also her co-workers, the manager, and the institution itself.

A few examples of enabling beliefs include the following:

- *Belief:* Getting treatment for the nurse will damage his career. Being treated for chemical dependency will be a permanent black mark on his personnel record. *Consequence:* Because the manager is too concerned about the nurse's career to see the threat to his life, she does nothing. She does not realize that referrals to treatment programs are confidential or that the disease and treatment programs are not mentioned in personnel records.
- *Belief:* Any nurse with an alcohol or other drug problem that affects job performance should be fired. *Consequence:* The nurse is fired, does not receive appropriate treatment, and the disease gets worse. If the nurse is employed at another hospital, the same set of problems recurs in a new environment. The nurse's dismissal also sends a message to other employees: "Keep quiet if you know someone who has a problem with alcohol or other drugs. You do not want to be blamed for getting someone fired."
- *Belief:* Taking any action is too painful, too difficult. It is better to leave things alone and hope that they will get better on their own or that the nurse will leave. *Consequence:* The problem does not remain static; it gets worse. And so does the nurse's condition. The pain for all concerned will progress along with the disease.
- *Belief:* The administration does not want managers to get involved in the nursing staff's personal problems. Perceived barriers in the system may include:
  − Complex disciplinary procedures[3]
  − Unsupportive upper-level managers[4]
  − Unsupportive union representatives[5]
  − Unclear performance standards[6]
  − Time constraints
  − Lack of proof that a problem exists
  − Fear of liability
  Consequence: No intervention takes place. Using system barriers (real or imagined) as excuses for failure to take action only

allows the situation to get worse. As the disease progresses and more staff members become involved, the risk to patient care increases and staff morale decreases. Eventually, the manager's effectiveness becomes impaired.

The following case history shows how easy it is for a manager to fall into an enabling posture. Nurse manager Pat Bixby eventually confronted Lois, a floor nurse, but only after a great deal of evidence had accumulated — and even then, the manager's tendencies toward enabling behavior threatened to intrude in the process.

"I can't believe it! She's my best nurse. I can't believe that she's been taking Demerol® from the unit. It just can't be. There has to be a mistake." The hospital pharmacist had just confronted the nurse manager on 7-West, a surgical floor, with documentation indicating that a large amount of Demerol® had been used on the unit in recent weeks. According to the controlled drug records, an unusually large quantity of Demerol® had been wasted, and there were no witnesses' signatures, as required by hospital policy, to document the losses. In addition, eight doses of Demerol® over a two-day period were signed out on the day shift as given to patients before the usual prescribed period of time between doses had elapsed. The data strongly indicated diversion of Demerol® from 7-West's controlled drug supply. From the evidence available, Lois, a nurse who had worked on 7-West for four years, was suspected.

Bixby was taken aback. How could this be? She had worked closely with Lois for the past four years. Surely, if there had been a problem, she would have known. She was aware that Lois had had some problems at home with her husband and problems with her own health. And Bixby acknowledged that she had occasionally been at the receiving end of Lois's mood swings. But she could always count on Lois to cover her shift and even work a double or extra shift on her day off when they were short-staffed.

In the past, when Bixby had attempted to discuss her concerns with Lois, Lois had always had an excuse and said, "Things will be okay. There's nothing to worry about." Despite Lois's personal problems, Bixby could not believe that she would ever steal drugs. She simply couldn't be an addict. Bixby's denial was very strong.

However, the pharmacist's documentation clearly pointed to a problem that needed immediate attention. Because Bixby was unable to dismiss the records and all the information that indicated Lois's involvement, she agreed with the pharmacist that they should meet with Lois to discuss the situation.

During the meeting, Lois vehemently denied any connection or involvement with the discrepancies. She lashed out at Bixby, accusing her of betraying their friendship, and was visibly angered and hurt. Even in light of the overwhelming documentation, Bixby began to feel that she might have made a mistake. But when Bixby continued to express her concern for Lois, Lois began to cry. She then asked to talk to Bixby alone.

When Bixby and Lois were alone, Lois broke down and told Bixby that she had been taking Demerol® for the past eight months. She was ashamed and contrite and agreed to get treatment for chemical dependency.

Later Bixby realized that she had almost withdrawn from the intervention when Lois denied her involvement. Despite the specific documentation and observable signs of job performance deterioration, Bixby had begun to question the evidence because of her relationship with Lois and her regard for her as a nurse.

Are You an Enabler?

Exercise 4-2 (on p. 65) can help nurse managers identify enabling attitudes and behaviors that potentially stand in the way of effective intervention. The rest of this book will address many of these issues. In addition, the appendix at the back of the book lists professional organizations for chemically dependent nurses and provides a list of suggested books and videos on chemical dependency. For more specific information and guidelines, nurse managers are encouraged to attend workshops on chemical dependency conducted by experts in the field or by professional organizations.

Achieving a true understanding of the disease of chemical dependency, however, takes time, patience, acceptance, and openness. Letting go of erroneous beliefs and enabling attitudes also takes time. Chemical dependency has been described over the years as "cunning and baffling." It is truly unique from other diseases nurses have studied and treated in their careers. Proficiency in identifying it—and dealing with it—should come with time and experience.

Hospitals and Other Health Care Institutions as Enablers

Most commonly, hospitals and other health care institutions act as enablers for chemically dependent nurses by failing to take appropriate measures rather than by taking deliberate actions. Examples of institutional enabling include the following:

- Health care institutions may lack specific policies and procedures related to alcohol and other drug use in the workplace and a philosophy that supports the institution's responsibility for its employees' well-being. Institutions may fail to have a policy that recognizes chemical dependency as a disease that can affect job performance and that supports the treatment of employees. Fitness-for-duty policies may also be neglected. Health care institutions may fail to develop specific procedures on intervention, referrals of nurses and other employees to treatment programs, and supervision during recovery. There may be no specific protocols in place for drug screening.

- Institutions may fail to provide educational programs on chemical dependency for all employees. Managers may not have been trained to identify the chemically dependent nurse and to intervene. Institutions may fail to provide consultation services for nurse managers.
- Health care institutions may provide inconsistent discipline for suspected alcohol and other drug users on staff. Without consistent implementation of disciplinary policies, other nurses may be afraid of the actions that the institution might take when a chemically dependent colleague's job performance becomes impaired. Thus, enabling behaviors increase and are reinforced.
- Health insurance coverage for the cost of appropriate treatment may be inadequate or nonexistent. Without reimbursement for substance abuse treatment services, chemically dependent nurses are unlikely to get the kind of treatment they need. Inadequate coverage sends the message that chemical dependency is not a disease requiring treatment, a message that further enables the dependent nurse.
- Health care institutions may not evaluate job performance on the basis of competency. Lack of routinely scheduled performance reviews with appropriate documentation and plans of action to correct deficiencies may make the identification of chemically dependent nurses more difficult.
- Health care institutions may not have an employee assistance program in place to assist nurse managers in the identification, referral, and treatment of chemically dependent nurses.
- Health care institutions may lack knowledge about resources and procedures for obtaining treatment for chemically dependent nurses. They also may lack information regarding intervention training and services.

How does your hospital rate on these points? If there is room for improvement, help get the institution on track. Discuss, educate, change. Seek out colleagues who support your commitment to change. (Chapter 10 of this book provides specific guidance.)

Universities and Other Schools of Nursing as Enablers

Schools for professional nursing education enable addicted nurses in many of the same ways that health care institutions do. In addition:

- They may fail to establish student assistance programs for identifying and referring student nurses to appropriate treatment facilities.
- Nursing programs may not offer comprehensive courses on chemical dependency as a part of the basic curriculum.
- Instructors may not be trained to identify, intervene, and arrange for the treatment of chemically dependent students.

Professionals as Enablers

Chemically dependent nurses may seek help from professionals voluntarily or at the urging of family, friends, or supervisors. When the professional is in the health care field, everyone assumes that she will be able to diagnose and treat the problem. However, not all health care professionals are familiar with the signs and symptoms of addiction, and many lack experience in treating chemical dependency.

Physicians

Nurses may consult physicians and receive treatment from them in all stages of the disease, including the early phases and recovery. Even in an effective doctor–patient relationship, however, the physician may actually enable the nurse's disease without realizing it. So may well-meaning but misguided physicians whom nurses encounter regularly in the hospital on a professional basis.

Physicians may enable chemically dependent nurses in the following ways:

- They may fail to obtain a comprehensive and reliable history of alcohol or other drug use from the nurse.
- They may lack education and knowledge about chemical dependency; that is, they may be unable to understand the nature and course of the disease, or they may fail to recognize its signs and symptoms.
- They may succumb to the chemically dependent nurse's manipulative behavior.
- They may inappropriately prescribe mood-altering chemicals.

- They may be too quick to medicate symptoms, going for the quick fix rather than conducting a thorough investigation to determine the nurse's primary problem.
- They may fail to refer nurses to specialists in the field of chemical dependency.
- They may assume a wait-and-see attitude in the hope that the nurse will realize that she has an alcohol or drug problem.
- They may allow the nurse to self-prescribe treatment.
- They may fail to give the nurse an honest diagnosis and prognosis.
- They may be unaware of resources for treatment and procedures for referral.

Mental Health Professionals

In an attempt to solve the problems brought on by their use of alcohol or other drugs, addicted nurses may enlist the services of mental health professionals, including counselors, social workers, and psychologists. When such professionals are not knowledgeable and experienced in chemical dependency treatment, however, further enabling is likely to occur. Enabling may result from any of the following:

- The mental health professional may lack thorough knowledge of chemical dependency and its treatment.
- The problem may be misdiagnosed, and inappropriate treatment may result.
- Mental health professionals may fail to accept chemical dependency as a primary disease.
- They may believe that the nurse will stop drinking or using drugs after he has solved his psychological problems.
- They may rely on individual psychotherapy in situations where group therapy is typically the treatment modality of choice because of the inherent support and confrontation among participants.
- They may continue treatment even after it has become apparent that the treatment is ineffective. The nurse keeps going to psychotherapy sessions but may do so under the influence of alcohol or other drugs or may refuse to work on issues related to her addiction. The therapist may mistakenly believe that the nurse is making progress because she continues to attend sessions.
- Mental health professionals may fail to include the nurse's family or significant others in the treatment program.

- They may believe mistakenly that the nurse may develop insights that eventually lead to a pattern of sensible substance use.

The Clergy

Clergy people are assumed to be caring, compassionate, and genuinely interested in the well-being of individuals. They provide guidance and comfort during times of stress and pain. Without knowledge and experience in chemical dependency, however, their interactions with chemically dependent nurses may be very enabling and actually promote the disease. For example:

- They may lack knowledge of the disease and nature of chemical dependency and its appropriate treatment.
- They may tend to deal with chemical dependency as a moral issue rather than as a treatable disease.
- They may rely exclusively on prayer as a solution.
- They may overemphasize the value of willpower in controlling addiction.
- They may try to "stay nice" and thereby fail to address the tough issues, or they may agree to keep the nurse's problem a secret.

To ensure that addicted nurses receive effective treatment, it is important to refer them to professionals or programs experienced in treating chemical dependency. (Suggested guidelines for making referrals are provided in chapter 6.)

Organizations as Enablers

Regulatory agencies such as state nursing boards and professional nursing associations also sometimes enable chemically dependent nurses through the organizations' lack of knowledge and understanding of chemical dependency. For example, in receiving complaints about incompetent nursing practice, nursing boards may take disciplinary action against nurses—direct them to take courses in medication documentation or the legal aspects of nursing, suspend their licenses, or place nurses on probation. Although these measures may be warranted in certain cases, rarely if ever is the issue of chemical dependency addressed. Consequently, upon meeting the condition(s) of the disciplinary action, the nurse returns to licensed practice even though he remains actively chemically dependent. Because he has not been referred for treatment, his practice remains compromised.

For example, Taylor, a 33-year-old registered nurse, was first reported to the Florida State Nursing Board by her employer in April 1975. The hospital had terminated her for making medication errors, incorrectly transcribing physicians' orders, and failing to chart properly. She found employment elsewhere but soon lost her job again for making medication errors. By April 1976, the nursing board had placed her on a two-year probation in response to the first employer's complaint.

Taylor was reinstated at the end of the probationary period and found work at a university hospital in the area. In September 1980, the hospital reported her to the nursing board for diverting Demerol® for her own use, administering Phenergan® to patients without a physician's authorization or knowledge, and charting Demerol® as having been administered to patients when in fact they had received a substitute. The nursing board suspended her license for one year and stipulated that she undergo psychiatric counseling, complete courses in charting and the legal aspects of nursing, and prove her competency to practice before being reinstated.

Taylor met the requirements and was placed on probation for two years. During the probationary period, she was investigated for, and admitted to, diverting Demerol® from the nursing home where she was employed at the time. The nursing home dismissed her in May 1983.

Subsequently, Taylor was admitted to a psychiatric unit for treatment of clinical depression. The state board accepted voluntary relinquishment of her license and ordered her to prove her ability to practice nursing safely before reinstatement.

She continued to receive outpatient psychiatric treatment and eventually began participating in a nurse support group. At a January 1986 support group meeting, the director of the state's newly formed Intervention Project for Nurses spoke to the members. In a conversation with Taylor, the director learned of her ongoing psychiatric treatment but discovered that she had never been treated for chemical dependency. Taylor was finally directed to an appropriate treatment program in 1986.[7]

Several state nursing boards have broken out of the enabling mode by developing diversion programs as an alternative to disciplinary action. These new programs are essentially monitoring, not treatment, programs. The program staff makes sure that nurses receive appropriate treatment, return to work only when they can do so safely, and make progress in recovery.

Florida became the first state to launch such an alternative program. The Impaired Nurses Program, now known as the Intervention Project for Nurses, was implemented in 1984 following the passage of state legislation in 1983. Through the project, nurses who have problems due to alcohol or drug abuse are referred for assessment and treatment of chemical dependency when appropriate. They are monitored by experienced chemical dependency nurses. A number of other states have started programs similar to Florida's. (The subject of alternative or diversion programs is discussed further in chapter 10.)

Professional nursing associations may also enable chemically dependent members through the lack of educational programs on chemical dependency in nursing and the lack of advocacy and peer assistance programs for addicted nurses. Another more subtle form of enabling is the lack of adequate reimbursement for chemical dependency treatment in association-sponsored group health plans.

Summary

Enabling is an example of the unique nature of chemical dependency as a disease. If a nurse were suffering from almost any other disease, friends, family, and co-workers would automatically urge him to seek care and treatment. Not so with chemical dependency. Often, the automatic response is to cover up for and protect the nurse—and thus perpetuate the disease. As a result, the disease "spreads," and those closest to the nurse suffer its effects as well.

Health care facilities, state nursing boards, and professional nursing associations may enable the addicted nurse further by failing to acknowledge the disease and develop policies, programs, and health insurance coverage to deal with it.

Because they are responsible for the care delivered by the nurses on their units, nurse managers can ill afford to enable chemically dependent nurses. But some do, for the reasons explained in this chapter. Once they identify their own enabling tendencies, however, they start freeing themselves from the web of enabling. When they do that, they are ready to put a stop to the human waste and suffering caused by chemical dependency among nurses.

☐ *References*

1. Krupnick, L., and Krupnick, E. *From Despair to Decision.* Minneapolis: CompCare Publications, 1985.
2. Wegscheider, S. *Another Chance.* Palo Alto, CA: Science and Behavior Books, 1981.
3. Blair, B. *Supervisors and Managers as Enablers,* rev. ed. Minneapolis: Johnson Institute, 1987.
4. Blair.
5. Blair.
6. Blair.
7. Penny, J. T., Catanzarite, A. M., and Ritter, J. K. Florida's alternative to disciplinary action. In: Haack, M. R., and Hughes, T. L., editors. *Addiction in the Nursing Profession.* New York City: Springer Publishing Co., 1989. [Case history adapted with permission.]

Exercise 4-1. Exploring the Manager's Attitudes
toward Chemical Dependency

On a sheet of paper, draw three columns, each with the following headings from left to right: Coronary Heart Disease Patient, Nurse, and Alcoholic/Addict. Then fill in the three columns by listing adjectives and verbs that reflect your ideas and feelings about each category of individual. Describe how you feel about each person and, in the case of the heart patient and the alcoholic/addict, what you want to do for them and how you respond to and feel about them.

Fill in the left column first and then the other two. Take time to probe your feelings. If you have trouble getting started, look at figure 4-2, which illustrates some attitudes other people have expressed. Try to come up with at least 5 to 10 words for each section.

What are the implications of this exercise? First, compare your responses in the left and right columns. Do they bear any similarity? Or were your responses quite different? If they were different, it is important for you to remind yourself that alcoholism and drug addiction are *chronic, progressive* diseases, much like coronary heart disease. Without treatment, the individual's condition advances, and early death becomes a real possibility. Addicts and alcoholics need empathy, appropriate treatment, education, reassurance, and support, just as coronary patients do. As with any disease, effective intervention and treatment of alcohol and drug addiction require a solid knowledge and understanding of the causes and effects of the illness.

Now, compare your responses in the center and right columns. Similar or different? Many nurse managers, like most people, have very negative feelings about alcoholics and addicts. Nurses, on the other hand, are seen as caring, helpful, and strong people. Because managers often regard alcoholics/addicts and nurses as exact opposites, it may be difficult for them to accept the fact that a nurse can be chemically dependent. Whenever a nurse is experiencing problems indicative of chemical dependency, the manager may simply deny that a problem exists. When both the manager and addicted nurse deny the problem, the disease worsens and intervention may never take place.

Figure 4-2. Examples of Attitudes toward Chemical Dependency

Coronary Heart Disease Patient	Nurse	Alcoholic/Addict
Afraid	Caring	"Skid row" bum
Sick	Kind	"Junkie"
In pain	Concerned	Weak
Care for	Dependable	Irresponsible
Educate	Responsible	Thief
Motivate	Stable	Out of control

Exercise 4-2. Identifying Enabling Attitudes and Behaviors

Place a check mark next to each statement that reflects your beliefs or behaviors.

_____ If a person really wants to stop drinking or using other drugs, all she needs to do is quit.

_____ I did not express my concern about another nurse who I felt had a problem with alcohol or other drugs because I was afraid of what his reaction might be.

_____ I have ignored inappropriate nursing behavior or denied suspicions of alcohol or other drug use.

_____ I believe that alcohol or other drug use in the workplace should be grounds for dismissal.

_____ I have covered up a nurse's alcohol or other drug use.

_____ I have failed to act on information pertaining to a nurse's drug use because I could not prove that he or she was chemically dependent.

_____ I believe that chemical dependency is a result of underlying psychological problems.

_____ I believe that my role and responsibility are to counsel employees who I believe may have a problem with alcohol or other drugs.

_____ I do not know how to obtain assistance for a nurse who has problems that may be related to alcohol or other drug use.

_____ I believe that chemical dependency is a sign of personal weakness.

_____ At times I have covered for nurses whom I suspected of chemical dependency and have assumed clinical responsibilities for them.

_____ I have refrained from getting involved or reporting my concerns for fear that the nurse would lose her job or license.

_____ I believe that good nurses do not become chemically dependent.

_____ I believe that it is necessary to diagnose the problem before referring a nurse to the employee assistance program.

_____ I have postponed taking action in the hope that things would get better and because I did not want to make waves.

_____ I do not understand how a chemically dependent nurse cannot see that he has a problem with alcohol or other drugs.

_____ I hesitate to ask a nurse to take a drug test because I do not want her to feel that I don't trust her.

_____ I believe that alcohol or other drug use is an individual's personal business and is not a concern of mine.

_____ I believe that a nurse must ask for help if she wants to get well.

Each of these is an enabling belief or behavior. If you discovered that you have some enabling tendencies, obtain additional knowledge and skills in how to deal with chemically dependent employees.

Documentation of the Signs and Symptoms of Chemical Dependency

At this point in the book, the nurse manager may be thinking:

> I can see how an individual's nursing practice is affected by her taking psychoactive, mood-altering drugs. I understand the difference between problem drinking or drug use and chemical dependency. I am also able to recognize the signs and symptoms of chemical dependency and have identified a nurse on the unit who may be addicted. I even realize how I may act as an enabler for a nurse who is chemically dependent. But where do I go from here?

Most nurse managers have access to specific information that will point to any problems that exist. It may be a history of absenteeism, declining standards of nursing care, discrepancies in medication records, inappropriate behavior, or similar signs and symptoms. Other staff members may have talked with the nurse manager about their concerns, complaints, and observations regarding the affected nurse.

At this point, the nurse manager is ready to document the signs and symptoms that have been identified. That is the focus of this chapter—how to establish specific documentation to support the manager's belief that a problem exists.

What Is Documentation?

Documenting the signs and symptoms of chemical dependency is a two-step process. The first step is gathering specific data and evidence to support the nurse manager's observations of inappropriate behavior in the workplace, employee complaints, concerns about impaired practice, and suspicions of chemical dependency. The second step involves recording the data and evidence along with the observations and complaints.

Gathering Data and Evidence

In gathering specific data and evidence, nurse managers have numerous sources to which they can refer, including nursing notes, controlled drug signout sheets, and personnel files. For example, a nurse's notes for a particular patient may be illogical or inappropriate for the patient's condition. Perhaps the patient received a medication that was not ordered by his physician. Attendance records in the nurse's personnel file are another good source of data. They may indicate that the nurse has been absent frequently without calling in or providing a plausible excuse.

Nurse managers who have only recently taken over their units and have noticed nursing problems should review existing written records. Managers who have supervised their units for some time and have observed some "problem nurses" but were unsure how to proceed should also review unit records. In both cases, the assumption is that the nurses in question have been chemically dependent for some time and have probably left a paper trail of discrepancies, declining job performance, and similar evidence behind them.

Some nurses, however, may have become problem drinkers or drug users only recently. They have not yet left a significant paper trail in nursing notes, controlled drug sheets, and personnel files. Managers should gather as many facts as possible about specific incidents of inappropriate or unprofessional behavior, find witnesses whenever possible, and record everything for later reference. If the incidents continue, a paper trail will probably soon emerge. The usual practice is to ask those staff members or other witnesses who come forward and express their concerns regarding the nurse in question to provide written, objective information on their observations. It is not appropriate for the nurse manager to question all employees to identify witnesses. In a facility where there are clearly defined policies and procedures and all employees have been educated to know that the facility supports assisting nurses who are experiencing problems and retaining them on staff, co-workers are more apt to come forward and express their concerns to the nurse managers.

Recording Data and Evidence

The second step in documentation involves recording the data and evidence in a confidential file that should be kept separate from the nurse's personnel file. The reason for keeping a separate file is that the nurse manager has not proved anything or taken any disciplinary action with respect to the nurse. The documentation file should be kept in a secure place where only the nurse manager has access to it. As new incidents occur or complaints surface, they should be documented and added to the file. In this way, the nurse manager can determine whether the incidents are one-time occurrences or elements of a pattern.

Why Document?

The documentation of signs and symptoms is essential for several reasons:

- Specific, factual information is needed to break through the nurse's wall of denial.
- The nurse manager must accept that objective information exists to support his concerns about the nurse. It is very easy for managers to attribute the signs and symptoms they have observed to something other than chemical dependency and so believe they have a rationale for not taking action. Enabling can be a very subtle process, and objective data help managers overcome their enabling tendencies.
- Legally, it may be necessary to substantiate that actions taken with respect to the nurse were based on facts, not innuendo or gossip. When the nurse is confronted during the intervention (see chapters 6 and 7), she may threaten to sue the health care facility. Objective facts and evidence can help defuse such threats, as well as serve as a defense in the event a lawsuit is actually filed in the future.

Documenting signs and symptoms is actually an important preliminary step to confronting the nurse with the reality of his situation. As mentioned earlier, nurses who are under the influence of alcohol or other drugs are unable to recognize that they have a problem. They are out of touch with what is really happening to them because of their strong denial. Specific data and evidence are vital in getting nurses to see the reality of their situation. Without specific data, an intervention is virtually impossible. The more thoroughly managers have documented a nurse's problem, the greater the likelihood that an intervention will succeed in getting the nurse to accept help.

As they gather documentation, managers should remember that they are not trying to diagnose the nurse's problem. They are simply gathering specific data to support the fact that there is a problem that must be addressed. In reviewing various records and files, they may uncover evidence that strongly suggests drug diversion, for example. Managers must refrain from making diagnoses, however, and leave that task to an addictions specialist.

When Should Documentation Be Started?

Evaluating the job performance of each nurse whom the manager supervises is an ongoing process. The manager is responsible for the care of patients on the unit, and this can best be achieved through the work of a qualified, competent, and healthy staff. The manager must also be responsive to problems that members of her staff are experiencing.

Typically, nurses experiencing problems due to alcohol or other drug use are unable to meet acceptable standards of patient care. Documentation therefore begins when an incident occurs that does not fall within acceptable standards of patient care, institutional policies and procedures, or appropriate professional behavior. The health care facility must take immediate steps to protect patients from the unsafe practice of chemically dependent nurses as soon as there is an indication that the nurse has a problem. This will also protect the institution from potential liability.

Each incident should be documented and addressed as it happens, whether it pertains to attendance, behavior, or job performance. It may turn out to be a one-time occurrence or the first in a long series of such incidents. If the incidents recur and the nurse does not respond to corrective action through traditional supervisory methods, an intervention must be planned. During the intervention, all the data and evidence collected earlier are laid out before the nurse by a team of caring colleagues who urge her to be evaluated and then treated, if necessary, for chemical dependency.

Managers frequently ask, "What should I do if I smell alcohol on the nurse's breath but do not see any other signs of a problem?" Alcohol on a nurse's breath is never acceptable in the workplace, whatever the reason. Some managers may act as enablers by explaining away the incident as simple overindulgence at a celebration. However, managers are not in a position to evaluate the extent of a nurse's drinking problem. After all, the nurse might be moving into the problem drinking stage, with such an incident being only the first manifestation of the problem in the workplace.

Managers should therefore document every incident and refer the nurse to the employee assistance program, employee health nurse, or a chemical dependency program for assessment. Early documentation and referrals may prevent the situation from advancing into full-blown addiction and impaired practice. (Chapter 10 presents specific policies and procedures for addressing the situations presented.)

How Is Documentation Accomplished?

As mentioned earlier in this chapter, gathering the specific data on which to base formal documentation of a problem involves identifying the data in written unit records and personnel files and gathering objective written accounts from witnesses. The accounts of witnesses are especially valuable when the nurse has not left a paper trail of evidence or when the nurse's behavior or performance has just become a noticeable problem.

Using Written Information

When a nurse has had a problem with alcohol or other drugs for some time, the nurse manager probably will be able to find evidence of the problem in various written records. Patient, unit, and personnel records often include strong evidence that a problem exists.

Patient Records

First, the nurse manager should review the nursing notes to make sure that they are appropriate and accurately reflect the care provided to patients and the progress or decline that patients have experienced. Incongruities are especially relevant, but any aberrations in the form or content of nursing notes can be used as documentation. The nurse manager should ask the following questions as she reviews a nurse's notes:

- Are the medications that patients received the ones physicians ordered?
- Are the notes complete and legible?
- Does the nurse's handwriting appear to get worse at any particular time during the shift?
- Do the nurse's notes accurately reflect the administration of controlled drugs and correspond with the controlled drug signout sheet?
- Do the notes reflect the patients' responses to analgesics?
- Are patients under the nurse's care complaining that their pain medication is not providing enough relief?
- Is the charting careless, with illogical entries?

The nurse manager should also look for other irregularities in patient medication records:

- Are patient medication records signed as required?
- Are the doses administered at the designated intervals and by the ordered route of administration?
- Do the signed doses correspond to those listed on the controlled drug signout sheet? To the nursing notes?

As managers review information in patient records, it is necessary to use other records to verify entries. For example:

- Does one nurse seem to administer more narcotics than the other nurses?
- Is there a physician's order for the medication apparently given?
- Is the correct dosage given at the ordered intervals?
- If a verbal order was taken, was it co-signed by the patient's physician during the required time frame?

Any entries or lack of entries in patient records that signal less than acceptable patient care or inaccurate or inappropriate charting should be recorded in the nurse's documentation file, but the file entries must be kept factual and nonjudgmental. For example:

Nurse reported on medication record that patient John Green received 100 mg Demerol® at 8:30 a.m. and 12:30 p.m., June 24, 1992. Nursing notes reflect same. But 100 mg Demerol® was signed out at 8:30 a.m., 11:00 a.m., and 12:30 p.m. on controlled drug sheet. No notation in nursing notes or patient's medication record that he received 11:00 a.m. dose. If he had received it, he would have been overmedicated. The doctor's order was for Demerol® every 3 to 4 hours as needed.

Unit Records

The unit records that provide managers with the most valuable information are the controlled drug signout sheets. Each nursing unit is responsible for documenting the administration of all controlled drugs allotted to that particular unit. The usual procedure is for each nurse to sign out each dose as it is given to the patient, indicating date, time, patient's name, and physician and including the nurse's signature to indicate that the drug was administered. Any wasted or spilled drugs and any broken containers must be appropriately accounted for and witnessed by a co-signer.

Any variations in adhering to these procedures should send up a red flag indicating the possibility that a staff member may have a drug problem. Incidents that suggest a problem include frequent wastages and breakages, unsigned drug administrations, lack of co-signatures when wastages occur, escalating drug supply needs for the unit, and overrepresentation of any one nurse in records of controlled drug administration.

Personnel Records

Nurse managers should review the nurse's personnel records. Incident/accident reports may indicate problems, for example:

- Does the nurse have an unusually high incidence of errors in practice and patient care?
- Do frequent accidents occur while the nurse is on duty?

Such incidents sometimes indicate problems due to inattention, impaired judgment, or lack of control caused by alcohol or other drug use.

Performance evaluations may demonstrate a decline in job performance. They may indicate job shrinkage as well—the nurse is doing less and not performing up to her prior level or even up to standards of acceptability. The nurse manager should ask:

- Does the nurse who welcomed new projects in the past now do only the minimum to get by?
- Does the performance evaluation indicate problems in getting along with co-workers or supervisors?
- Does the evaluation indicate that there have been problems with patients and their families?

The nurse's prior work history may provide additional information. For example:

- Has the nurse (or his managers) requested frequent transfers within the institution?
- Did former employers provide favorable references?
- Did former employers say that they would reemploy the nurse?
- Did the nurse provide appropriate explanations for any periods of unemployment on the employment application?

- Does the nurse appear to job-hop; that is, are there numerous periods of employment of one year or less?
- What reasons has the nurse given for changing employers?
- Are there any disciplinary actions on the nurse's employment record?
- Has the nurse been disciplined by her current employer or by the state board of nursing?
- What reasons were given for any disciplinary action?
- Have the conditions that prompted disciplinary action in the past been corrected, or are the same problems, behaviors, or situations recurring?

Attendance records can also provide specific data that indicate a problem. For example:

- Does the nurse take an unusually high number of sick days?
- Do the absences occur at particular times, perhaps after holidays or weekends?
- Are there frequent unexcused absences or improbable excuses for absences?
- Does the nurse call in sick at the last minute or not at all?
- Is the nurse frequently absent from his assigned unit when on duty?
- Does the nurse head for the restroom or leave the unit after accessing the controlled drug cabinet?
- Is the nurse frequently confused about the work schedule?
- Is the opposite of absenteeism occurring? Does the nurse frequently appear on the unit on days off?

In addition, managers may be aware of legal problems the nurse is experiencing, including arrests or citations for driving under the influence (DUI) or driving while intoxicated (DWI); family problems such as separation or divorce; domestic violence; child abuse; problems with children such as running away and delinquency; or financial problems.

A typical documentation file entry based on the manager's review of the nurse's personnel record might read as follows:

Five documented instances of complaints from patients' family members in the last month alone. Reports specified that nurse was short-tempered with patients Green, Taylor, Moore, Celli, and Martin.

Gathering Data When No Supporting Written Information Is Available

If a nurse is just beginning to have problems with alcohol or other drugs, there may be little or no supporting written data in patient, unit, or personnel records. Her performance and work record may have been exemplary in the past. The very first indication of a problem may be liquor on the nurse's breath, a staggering gait, or a decline in appearance. How should nurse managers go about documenting incidents like these?

The best procedure to follow is this:

- Record as many specifics as possible, including when the incident took place, what happened, who was involved, and what the nurse's reactions and behaviors were.
- Find witnesses to the incident whenever possible and have them record objectively what they observed.
- Explain any problems the behavior caused. This is important because chemically dependent nurses deny that their use of alcohol or drugs is causing problems. For example, the nurse manager might document having smelled liquor on a nurse's breath in the following way:

    On May 6, 1992, when nurse Jones reported for duty, I smelled liquor on her breath. When she entered the nurses' station, she was unsteady, stumbled into the chair, and used the wall behind to steady herself. When I attempted to help, she pushed me away and said, "I'm OK. I don't need your help." Her speech was slurred and it was difficult to understand her. Jackie Mills and John Cameron were in the nurses' station at the time and tried to help. She pushed them away as well.

(In this situation, in addition to documentation, the nurse should be immediately evaluated for her fitness for duty. See chapter 10.)

Because other staff members witnessed this incident, the manager asked them to write a description of what they saw in the same objective manner. Their accounts were added to the documentation file. In writing down what they saw, staff members were not "ganging up" or "ratting" on the nurse, but documenting specific behaviors that indicate the nurse needs help. However, the nurse manager must be careful about what she says to other staff members because she might be liable for slander if she makes any charges that later prove false or misrepresented. Staff must report objective information only, not their personal conclusions, feelings, or beliefs pertaining to the incident.

Documentation Exercises

Real-life incidents in which documentation played a key role in substantiating nurses' alcohol or drug use problems are useful learning tools, as in exercises 5-1 and 5-2, beginning on p. 78. (Names have been changed to protect patients' confidentiality and nurses' true identities.) The documentation gathered from drug and patient records in these cases was later used to successfully intervene with the nurses involved.

Each exercise requires the reader to perform a chart audit. Sample records, shown in the figures, are examined before pertinent questions are answered. At the end of each example, the correct answers will be reviewed.

Chart audits in which controlled drug signout sheets, patient medication records, nursing notes, and physicians' orders are reviewed can be extremely helpful in documenting diversion. Nurse managers can also use the same procedures when they are not aware of any drug discrepancies but are concerned about a nurse's declining job performance and behavior. Very often, the results of the audit will help document a problem and provide additional valuable information for conducting an effective intervention.

Summary

Documenting the signs and symptoms of chemical dependency is a two-step process. Managers gather specific data and evidence to support observations and complaints about the nurse and then record the information in a special documentation file. The file is kept separate from the nurse's personnel record, in a secure place where only the manager can gain access to it.

There are two basic techniques for gathering data and evidence. In the first, managers review patient, unit, and personnel records. They may discover drug discrepancies, job-hopping tendencies, inappropriate charting, or erratic handwriting, among other things. In the second, managers gather as many facts as possible and get witnesses to substantiate observations and complaints against the nurse. Managers typically use this technique when they are just beginning to notice a problem with the nurse or when the nurse only recently began having problems. In the latter case, there is often no paper trail of written information in patient, unit, or personnel records.

It is well worth the effort to document signs of chemical dependency. The specific factual data gathered in the process help break through the nurse's denial during an intervention. Objective documentation also helps overcome any enabling tendencies in the manager. In addition, it is a sound legal practice.

Managers should start documentation when the first incident occurs that falls outside acceptable practice standards, institutional policies and procedures, or appropriate behavior. They should also address those issues according to customary supervisory policies and procedures. Even the first instance of alcohol on the breath, slurred speech, or staggering gait warrants documentation and a referral for professional help at once.

Exercise 5-1. Documentation Exercise 1

On June 30, 1991, at the change of shift on 4E, a surgical unit, the narcotic count for Demerol® 100 mg is correct. Of the allotted 25 Tubex® doses, 16 remain. The narcotic count corresponds to the controlled drug signout sheet (see figure 5-1).

First, examine figure 5-1 in detail. Is everything in order? Have normally accepted procedures been followed? Do you see any problems or discrepancies of any kind? If so, what? (Write your answers on a separate sheet of paper.)

Next, review figure 5-2 (patient George's medication record) and figure 5-3 (patient George's nursing notes). After reviewing all three records pertaining to patient George, answer the following questions:

- What is the situation as you now see it?
- Are there any discrepancies or abnormalities? If so, what are they?
- What possible conclusion could you draw from your analysis?

Now, review the patient and unit records together. In general, the controlled drug signout sheet seems to be in order. The 16 Tubex® *syringes of Demerol®* 100 mg on hand correspond to the control sheet. Each individual dose is appropriately signed for by a nurse. However, there is a red flag! Patient George's 9 a.m. dose was apparently given to him 2½ hours after the 6:30 a.m. dose. Usually, Demerol® is given every 3 to 4 hours. Further investigation is warranted.

The doses signed out to patient George at 9 a.m. and 12 p.m. apparently were not given to him. There is no corresponding documentation on his medication record or nursing notes. In fact, he was not on 4E at the time, but in surgery and then the recovery room. Patient George left 4E at 6:50 a.m. for surgery and returned to his room at 2:15 p.m. Nurse S. Griffin signed out the doses at 9 a.m. and 12 noon, apparently for Mr. George. Yet he never received them.

If you said that S. Griffin possibly diverted the Demerol® you are correct. The discrepancies identified can be attributed to her. In reality, this information was discovered when a chart audit was conducted because of complaints from co-workers about the nurse. Co-workers noted her irritability, inappropriate behavior, and inattention to patient requests. By conducting an audit of patient George's records, the nurse manager obtained valuable documentation that was effectively used in the intervention with nurse Griffin.

Because the initial narcotic count in this case appeared to be correct, how likely is it that the drug diversion would have been detected? The red flag raised by the shortened interval of Demerol® administration prompted further investigation. Are routine audits of controlled drugs conducted on your unit?

Figure 5-1. Controlled Drug Signout Sheet (for Exercise 5-1)

CONTROL NO.
23392

CONTROL NO.

MFG. CONTROL NO.: _____ EXPIRES: _____ SHEET RETURNED: _____
DRUG: DEMEROL INJ STRENGTH: 100 mg QUANTITY: 25
ISSUED BY: BILL JERI RPh TO STATION: 4E DATE ISSUED: 6/29/91
RECEIVED BY: ANN GOODMAN RN (NURSE IN CHARGE) DATE: 6/29/91

BAL	DATE	TIME	PATIENT'S NAME	ROOM NO.	PHYSICIAN	DOSE	ADMINISTERED BY
25	6/30/91	6³⁰ AM/PM	GEORGE, T.	428	BRUCE	100mg	A. Goodman RN
24	6/30/91	7⁰⁰ AM/PM	TAYLOR, R.	422	SHAMP	100 mg	K. Lee RN
23	6/30/91	7³⁰ AM/PM	MARCUS, P.	421	KELT	100 mg	B. Smith RN
22	6/30/91	8⁴⁵ AM/PM	JERUSO, M.	418	GREENE	100 mg	T. Kelly RN
21	6/30/91	9⁰⁰ AM/PM	GEORGE, T.	428	BRUCE	100 mg	S. Griffin RN
20	6/30/91	11³⁵ AM/PM	TAYLOR, R.	422	SHAMP	100mg	K. Lee RN
19	6/30/91	12⁰⁰ AM/PM	GEORGE, T.	428	BRUCE	100 mg	S. Griffin RN
18	6/30/91	2⁴⁵ AM/PM	MARCUS, P.	421	KELT	100 mg	B. Smith RN
17	6/30/91	3⁰⁰ AM/PM	GEORGE, T.	428	BRUCE	100 mg	S. Griffin RN
16		AM/PM					
15		AM/PM					
14		AM/PM					
13		AM/PM					
12		AM/PM					
11		AM/PM					
10		AM/PM					
9		AM/PM					
8		AM/PM					
7		AM/PM					
6		AM/PM					
5		AM/PM					
4		AM/PM					
3		AM/PM					
2		AM/PM					
1		AM/PM					

Figure 5-1. (Continued)

RECORD OF WASTE AND SPOILAGE

ITEM	DATE	QUANTITY	DESCRIBE IN DETAIL	SIGNATURE NO. 1	SIGNATURE NO. 2

I hereby certify that the above doses were given as per written order by a physician on the treatment sheets of the above-named patients.

DATE RETURNED: _____ SIGNED: _____
(Supervisor)

Figure 5-2. Patient George's Medication Record

Initials	Full Signature	Title	Initials	Full Signature	Title
ag	*Anne Goodman*	RN			
SG	*Susan Griffin*	RN			
Initials	Full Signature	Title	Initials	Full Signature	Title

PRN Medications   PRN's should also be recorded in nurse's notes

OR DATE INITIALS	EXP. DATE TIME	MEDICATION-DOSAGE-FREQUENCY RT. OF ADM.		DOSES GIVEN						
		Demerol 100 mg *Inj.* *q 3-4 hr prn*	DATE	6/30	6/30					
			TIME	6:30 am	3 pm					
			INIT	*ag*	*SG*					
			DATE							
			TIME							
			INIT							
			DATE							
			TIME							
			INIT							
			DATE							
			TIME							
			INIT							
			DATE							
			TIME							
			INIT							
			DATE							
			TIME							
			INIT							
			DATE							
			TIME							
			INIT							
			DATE							
			TIME							
			INIT							
			DATE							
			TIME							
			INIT							
			DATE							
			TIME							
			INIT							

Figure 5-3. Patient George's Nursing Notes

CLINICAL RECORD MIDNIGHT TO MIDNIGHT		NURSE'S NOTES
DATE AND HOUR	DRUGS, DRESSINGS, TRAYS AND SPECIALTY TREATMENT	OBSERVATIONS (when indicated include intake and output, type, amount, and time)
6/30/91 4am		patient sleeping a. Goodman RN
5³⁰ am		patient awake V/S B/P 120/70 P-84, R-16, T 98.4° prepared for abdominal surgery a. Goodman RN
6³⁰ am	Demerol 100 mg Valium 10 mg	IM (R) hip ⟩ preops per IM (R) hip ⟩ order a. Goodman RN
6⁵⁰ am		pt. to OR. family present. PT appears to be sleeping comfortably. a. Goodman RN
2¹⁵ pm		Pt. returns to Rm. 428 from RR. Awake - V/S stable. B/P 120/80, P 90, R 16, T 99.4°. Appears comfortable. S. Griffin RN
3 pm	Demerol 100 mg	IM (L) hip as requested for pain in operative area. S. Griffin RN
3¹⁵ pm		appears comfortable. Family present. S. Griffin RN

Exercise 5-2. Documentation Exercise 2

The entire allotment of 25 Tubex® doses of Demerol® 100 mg has been used for patients in the coronary care unit. The controlled drug signout sheet is ready to be returned to the pharmacy, and the unit will be restocked. Review figure 5-4 (the controlled drug signout sheet).

- Is everything in order?
- Do you have any questions?
- Are there any discrepancies?
- If so, what are they?

Next, review figures 5-5 (patient Moore's medication record) and 5-6 (patient Taylor's medication record). Answer the following questions:

- What did you discover about patient Taylor and patient Moore with respect to medication administration?
- Is there any one nurse you're concerned about in light of the information you have documented?
- From the records, how many 100-mg doses of Demerol® appear to have been diverted, that is, how many are unaccounted for?
- When were the doses apparently diverted?
- What conclusion might you draw from the information you have gathered?

Now, let's review the records together. Figure 5-4 (the controlled drug signout sheet) raises some questions about the frequency of dosage administration. It appears that some doses were given within a shorter interval of time than normal. For example:

- Patient Taylor was given a dose at 8:10 a.m. and again at 10:03 a.m. on 6/26, at an interval of less than 2 hours.
- Patient Moore was given a dose at 10:15 a.m. and again at 11:30 a.m. on 6/25, at an interval of 1 hour, 15 minutes. After the dose he received at 11:30 a.m., he received another at 1:48 p.m. at an interval of 2 hours, 18 minutes. On the next day, 6/26, he was given a dose at 7:00 a.m. and again at 9:05 a.m., at an interval of 2 hours, 5 minutes. After the 9:05 a.m. dose, he received another at 10:20 a.m., at an interval of 1 hour, 15 minutes.

All the entries in question were charted as administered by nurse E. Jackson.

After reviewing patient Taylor's medication record, we discover that the 10:03 a.m. dose on 6/26 is not charted on the record. The physician's order specifies that Demerol® is to be given every 3 to 4 hours. If the patient had received the 10:03 a.m. dose, it would have been given within less than a two-hour interval. Patient Moore's medication record does not indicate that he received the 11:30 a.m. dose on 6/25 or the 9:05 a.m. and 10:20 a.m. doses on 6/26. Also, the doses recorded as having been given at 10:20 a.m. and 1:48 p.m. on 6/26 were administered within a shorter interval than ordered.

If your concern was about nurse E. Jackson, you are correct. All the questionable medication administrations were signed by him. From the records, it appears that four doses, or 400 mg, of Demerol® were diverted and that the doses in question were obtained on 6/25 at 11:30 a.m. and on 6/26 at 9:05, 10:03, and 10:20 a.m. From all the information provided, it appears that nurse Jackson falsified patient records and possibly diverted the drugs in question to himself.

Figure 5-4. Controlled Drug Signout Sheet (for Exercise 5-2)

CONTROL NO.

23392

CONTROL NO.

MFG. CONTROL NO.: _____ EXPIRES: _____ SHEET RETURNED: _____
DRUG: Demerol Inj STRENGTH: 100 mg QUANTITY: 25
ISSUED BY: Green RPh TO STATION: CCU DATE ISSUED: 6/25/91
RECEIVED BY: Evan Jackson RN (NURSE IN CHARGE) DATE: 6/25/91

BAL	DATE	TIME	PATIENT'S NAME	ROOM NO.	PHYSICIAN	DOSE	ADMINISTERED BY
25	6/25	9⁰⁵ AM	Taylor	568	Dillon	100	E. Jackson
24	6/25	10¹⁵ AM	Moore	561	Moore	100	Jackson
23	6/25	11⁰¹ AM	Smith	560	Tucker	100	Williams
22	6/25	11³⁰ AM	Moore	561	Mills	100	Jackson
21	6/25	11³⁵ AM	Caruso	562	Jones	100	Williams
20	6/25	1¹⁰ PM	Andrews	563	Jones	100	Kelly
19	6/25	1⁴⁵ AM	Taylor	568	Dillon	100	Jackson
18	6/25	1⁴⁸ PM	Moore	561	Mills	100	Jackson
17	6/25	3¹⁰ AM	Brown	567	Gates	100	Warren
16	6/25	6³⁰ PM	Caruso	562	Jones	100	Black
15	6/25	7¹⁵ AM	Smith	560	Tucker	100	Williams
14	6/25	9³⁵ AM	Taylor	568	Dillon	100	Hope
13	6/25	11⁰⁰ AM	Moore	561	Mills	100	Hope
12	6/26	1¹⁰ PM	Brown	567	Gates	100	Parrish
11	6/26	3⁴⁰ AM	Moore	561	Mills	100	Hope
10	6/26	7⁰⁰ AM	Moore	561	Mills	100	Jackson
9	6/26	8¹⁰ PM	Taylor	568	Dillon	100	Jackson
8	6/26	9⁰⁵ AM	Moore	561	Mills	100	Jackson
7	6/26	9⁰⁷ PM	Smith	560	Tucker	100	Jackson
6	6/26	10⁰³ PM	Taylor	568	Dillon	100	Jackson
5	6/26	10¹⁵ PM	Brown	567	Gates	100	Warren
4	6/26	10²⁰ AM	Moore	561	Mills	100	Jackson
3	6/26	12¹⁵ PM	Smith	560	Tucker	100	Jackson
2	6/26	12³⁰ AM	Moore	561	Mills	100	Jackson
1	6/26	1⁵⁵ PM	Caruso	562	Jones	100	Black

Figure 5-4. (Continued)

RECORD OF WASTE AND SPOILAGE

ITEM	DATE	QUANTITY	DESCRIBE IN DETAIL	SIGNATURE NO. 1	SIGNATURE NO. 2

I hereby certify that the above doses were given as per written order by a physician on the treatment sheets of the above-named patients.

DATE RETURNED: _____ SIGNED: _____
                                            (Supervisor)

Figure 5-5. Patient Moore's Medication Record

Initials	Full Signature	Title	Initials	Full Signature	Title
EJ	*E. Jackson*	RN			
J.H.	*J. Hope*	RN			
Initials	Full Signature	Title	Initials	Full Signature	Title

PRN Medications   PRN's should also be recorded in nurse's notes

OR DATE INITIALS	EXP. DATE TIME	MEDICATION-DOSAGE-FREQUENCY RT. OF ADM.		DOSES GIVEN							
		Demerol 100 IM	DATE	6/25	6/25	6/25	6/26	6/26	6/26		
		q 4h prn	TIME	10⁸	1⁴⁵	11⁰⁰ P	3⁴⁰ A	7⁰⁰ A	12³⁰ P		
			INIT	EJ	EJ	JH	JH	EJ	EJ		
			DATE								
			TIME								
			INIT								
			DATE								
			TIME								
			INIT								
			DATE								
			TIME								
			INIT								
			DATE								
			TIME								
			INIT								
			DATE								
			TIME								
			INIT								
			DATE								
			TIME								
			INIT								
			DATE								
			TIME								
			INIT								
			DATE								
			TIME								
			INIT								

Figure 5-6. Patient Taylor's Medication Record

Initials	Full Signature	Title	Initials	Full Signature	Title
EJ	E. Jackson	RN			
EW	E. Williams	RN			
MK	M. Kelly	RN			
MW	M. Warren	RN			
JH	J. Hope	RN			
Initials	Full Signature	Title	Initials	Full Signature	Title

PRN Medications   PRN's should also be recorded in nurse's notes

OR DATE INITIALS	EXP. DATE TIME	MEDICATION-DOSAGE-FREQUENCY RT. OF ADM.		DOSES GIVEN							
		Demerol 100 mg IM q 3-4 hrs	DATE	6/25	6/25	6/25	6/26				
			TIME	9:05A	1:45P	9:35P	8:10A				
			INIT	EJ	EJ	JH	EJ				
			DATE								
			TIME								
			INIT								
			DATE								
			TIME								
			INIT								
			DATE								
			TIME								
			INIT								
			DATE								
			TIME								
			INIT								
			DATE								
			TIME								
			INIT								
			DATE								
			TIME								
			INIT								
			DATE								
			TIME								
			INIT								
			DATE								
			TIME								
			INIT								

Preparation for an Intervention

"To wait for an individual who is chemically dependent to ask for help is like waiting for an individual who is unconscious after a myocardial infarction to ask for help."[1] Health care professionals do not wait for people having myocardial infarctions (MI) to ask for help because they are unable to ask for help. Instead, cardiopulmonary resuscitation (CPR) is initiated immediately. The chemically dependent nurse is just as unable to ask for help as an MI patient. Because of her continual denial and the delusional nature of chemical dependency, the nurse is unaware of her disease. The response must be the same, that is, CPR (concerned people responding).[2] Health care professionals must intervene in both situations because they are dealing with life-threatening diseases in both situations.

Nurses use intervention techniques every day. In doing so, their intent is clearly to interrupt a debilitating and often life-threatening situation—to stop a destructive, deteriorating process. They intervene with patients and their families in order to heal, comfort, and protect.

The process of intervening with a chemically dependent nurse, however, is a new idea for most nurse managers, and one that often produces anxiety and concern. This chapter and the next focus on the process of intervening with chemically dependent nurses. Chapter 6 explains what an intervention is, when to decide that an intervention is necessary, and how to prepare for one. Chapter 7 describes an actual intervention to illustrate the process.

A Definition of Intervention

When a nurse manager intervenes with a nurse who is suspected of being chemically dependent, the goal is to get the nurse to accept help. It is also hoped that he will get appropriate treatment, begin recovery, and live life free from the devastation of alcohol and other drugs. Still, these anticipated results are outside the nurse manager's control; no one can be forced into recovery. What nurse managers can do is confront the nurse with specific information about the apparent problem and direct and assist her toward appropriate evaluation and treatment.

The most effective definition of the term *intervention* was developed by the man who originated the process, Vernon Johnson, D.D. Johnson defined it as "the presentation of reality to a person who is out of touch with it, in a receivable way."[3] By a "presentation of reality," Johnson means a presentation of specific facts regarding the chemically dependent person's behavior and its effects. By "in a receivable way," he means that the facts should be presented in a direct, objective, nonjudgmental, and caring way. Accusations and complaints have no place in an intervention.

Helping the nurse to see and accept reality is crucial to the intervention process. Because of all the chaos and unmanageability in a chemically dependent nurse's life, he is out of touch with reality, which makes it impossible for him to see that alcohol or other drugs are the problem.

The participants in an intervention confront the nurse's denial by focusing on examples of her inappropriate behavior. An intervention is not a personal attack on the nurse; it is a structured process to confront the effects of the disease. This approach usually works, and in the vast majority of cases, the nurse agrees to accept evaluation and treatment.

Ultimately, intervention is the only way to break the addiction cycle. If the nurse were dismissed instead, she would go on to another job, where the same plot would eventually unfold. Chemically dependent nurses enter treatment more willingly when they have a job they want to keep and have the medical benefits that cover the cost of treatment. When they are between jobs or on a new job before benefits become effective, they are less likely and less able to enter treatment because they do not have the financial resources to do so. The health care facility also benefits from intervention, because chemical dependency is a treatable disease from which the nurse can recover and subsequently return to competent practice.

The person responsible for initiating the intervention is the nurse manager, because the manager is accountable for the patient care provided by nurses on the unit. By the time a nurse shows signs of chemical dependency, nursing care is compromised and patients are put at risk. Managers are also responsible for providing a safe work environment for their staff. Often, co-workers end up taking over the chemically dependent nurse's duties as the disease worsens. Eventually, they feel used, frustrated, resentful, and tired, and their performance, in turn, is affected. It is clearly the manager's responsibility to intervene and stop the disease from affecting those who work with and are cared for by the nurse. Morale declines dramatically when the nurse manager fails to take action.

Some Common Misconceptions about Intervention

Because most nurse managers lack experience in intervening with chemically dependent nurses, they may bring some misconceptions to the first few interventions. Three of the most common misconceptions are these — that in order for the intervention to be successful:

- The nurse manager needs proof that the nurse is chemically dependent, that is, that the problem is attributable to problems with alcohol or other drugs.
- The manager needs to break down the nurse's defensive denial.
- The nurse must admit or confess to diverting drugs, drinking on the job, or doing something similar.

The Need for Proof

Proof of chemical dependency is *not* necessary before an intervention can take place. Typically, the manager has observed clear signs that the nurse's practice is impaired or below standard. Even when the nurse's practice has not yet been noticeably affected, there are still behavioral signs or physical manifestations that are not appropriate to the workplace. An intervention is called for whether or not the cause of the signs and symptoms is chemical dependency. Nurse managers are expected to know when there is a problem in meeting professional standards. They are not expected to know the cause, and they are not responsible for diagnosing the problem and then proving the accuracy of the diagnosis. Nurse managers are responsible, however, for intervening to put a stop to the problem and address its causes.

Managers who feel that they need proof often wait until they "catch" the nurse with a needle in his arm or a shot of vodka in her coffee. At that stage, the disease is advanced, and the dangers to the nurse, the patients, and the workplace are great. Patients are at risk of compromised care, and co-workers have become so enmeshed in the nurse's dysfunction that their practice and behaviors are often affected. Intervention may be successful at this stage but should have been attempted much earlier with the information available. It is not necessary to catch the nurse or to know what is causing the dysfunction in order to take appropriate action.

The Need to Pierce Denial

The intervention team may believe that it must break through the nurse's denial and make the nurse acknowledge that alcohol or other drugs are a problem for her. However, this is not the team's job, and this most often does not occur until the nurse undergoes treatment. What frequently happens during an intervention is that the nurse thinks that the team is all wrong and, to prove it, agrees to an evaluation for chemical dependency. Even when the evaluation indicates dependency, the nurse very often insists that the evaluation is wrong. Often, the nurse enters treatment because she is concerned about losing her job or license but remains in denial. This situation should be perfectly acceptable to the team; after all, the goal is getting the nurse to agree to evaluation and treatment. The initial objective of treatment is to pierce denial and to help the nurse accept that he has a disease and realize that he is powerless over alcohol or other drugs.

The Need to Obtain an Admission of Guilt

Another misconception is that the intervention team must get the nurse to admit to errors or deceptions, such as diverting drugs, or to identify herself as an alcoholic. If this were the team's goal, the team would probably have to wait forever. When a team insists on getting the nurse to admit or confess, the nurse usually becomes resentful, denies the problem even more vigorously, and refuses to accept help at all. Strong emotions are aroused, and the nurse feels as though she is being backed into a corner. The team's sole job is to get the nurse to agree to seek help, not to get the nurse to admit or confess guilt. The evaluation and treatment program staff will help the nurse to recognize her problems and deceptions.

Nurse managers often feel concerned, confused, and frustrated if they cannot get the nurses involved to admit to all the incidents with which they are confronted. This occurs because so much of a manager's role involves problem solving. In cases concerning chemical dependency or other mental health issues, however, the manager's role is only to intervene and assist the nurse in accepting help.

The Decision to Act

Nurse managers frequently ask the question, "How much information do I need before I can intervene?" They are often at a loss to determine when to act, which goes back to their erroneous assumption that they must be able to prove chemical dependency before they can act. Clearly, a manager has enough information when he sees behaviors, attitudes, or actions in the workplace that are contrary to acceptable nursing practice. It may take a while for managers to recognize the signs and symptoms of chemical dependency, but all managers know what constitutes competent nursing care and appropriate behavior in the health care workplace.

Usually, a specific incident causes the manager to say, "Enough! This has to stop. It cannot continue!" Very often, the manager reaches this point after other attempts to correct the problem have failed. The triggering incident may be an unexcused absence, an outburst of anger toward a co-worker, an incorrect narcotics count, or a staff member's complaint. It may be the same old behavior or some new, more serious behavior that pushes the manager to say, "This must stop!" The next logical step is intervention.

Unclear or nonexistent policies and procedures for dealing with chemically dependent employees can thwart a manager's resolve to intervene, however. One manager had documented a nurse's increasing absenteeism, negative attitude, and failure to meet deadlines. Even though she had sufficient information to conduct an intervention with an expectation of success, she became confused and frustrated when she consulted with the employee health nurse and was told to get more conclusive information — in essence, to *prove* the cause of the problem. Consequently, she backed off from holding an intervention, and the employee's condition continued to deteriorate.

In this case, the hospital lacked clear policies and procedures for dealing with staff who may be abusing alcohol or other drugs or exhibiting problems in the workplace. Moreover, staff members whom nurse managers would likely consult about chemical dependency problems had varying degrees of education and expertise in handling addictions. This was clearly an enabling situation. A concerned manager who wanted to take effective action was thwarted in her attempt because of an enabling administrative system. She, and managers like her, need to work for change within their facilities. (Chapter 10 provides guidance on how to set up an effective in-house drug and alcohol program.)

Steps in the Intervention Process

The intervention process involves a number of steps, several of which are preparatory and take place in advance of the actual intervention. Thorough preparation is essential to a successful outcome. At first, preparation will take a fair amount of the manager's time. After the manager gains experience and confidence, preparation time significantly decreases. As was indicated earlier, the nurse manager is assumed to be the person responsible for doing all the preparation for the intervention. Some of these steps may be facilitated by an EAP counselor, a psychiatric nurse liaison, or other identified individual to provide assistance or consultation.

Major steps in the intervention process are the following:

1. Document the signs, symptoms, and incidents as closely as possible.
2. Select the intervention team.
3. Identify the financial resources available for treatment.
4. Identify treatment programs.
5. Meet with the intervention team. The team should accomplish the following:
   — Review key facts about chemical dependency.
   — Develop scripts for the intervention on the basis of firsthand information that each team member has gathered on the nurse's behaviors and performance.
   — Agree on a plan of action that the team will ask the nurse to accept.
   — Assign team members to the roles they will play and the tasks they will perform during the intervention.
   — Make contingency plans. Review possible scenarios of what could happen during the intervention so that the team will be prepared to act fast if necessary.
   — Rehearse the intervention.
   — Set a time and place for the intervention.
   (Because there is so much preparation work, the manager may want to divide the tasks among two [or more] meetings — perhaps tasks 1 through 4 in one meeting, and the rest in another. If the need to intervene is immediate, preparation time can and must be significantly reduced.)
6. Conduct the intervention.

No two interventions are exactly alike. They vary with the personalities involved, the stage of chemical dependency, how knowledgeable the team is about the disease, the extent of health insurance coverage, and other factors.

If the team follows the plan outlined in this chapter, however, its chances of succeeding will be at least 80 percent.[4] Many believe the success ratio to be even higher for health care professionals because of the leverage that can be brought to bear on them and their fears about maintaining their professional status and licensure.

Step One: Document the Signs, Symptoms, and Incidents

As discussed in chapter 5, the first step in preparing for the intervention is the documentation of the signs and symptoms that suggest that a nurse may have a drug or alcohol problem. Specific incidents should be described and, if possible, eyewitness accounts should be included in the documentation file.

Step Two: Select the Intervention Team

After documenting the nurse's behavior and/or incidents of impaired practice, the manager is ready to select the intervention team. Interventions are never conducted one-on-one between the nurse and the nurse manager. When the nurse manager alone confronts the nurse with specific information, it is very easy for the nurse to dismiss the manager's concerns and view the whole confrontation as a personal attack. A one-on-one confrontation simply is not powerful enough to deal with the disease of chemical dependency.

A team intervention during which several people present data to the nurse has greater impact. The minimum number recommended for an intervention team is two. There is no maximum, but it is a good idea to keep the team at a workable number, usually four or five. Maintaining control during the intervention is very important, and too many people make maintaining control difficult. However, determining who should be on the team is more important than deciding the number of participants.

Two people belong on the team automatically by virtue of their positions:

- *The nurse manager,* who has a close working relationship with the nurse and is directly responsible for the nurse's supervision. The manager has collected specific information on inappropriate behaviors and should be the one to present the information during the intervention.
- *Another authority figure,* usually the director of nursing, an administrator, or a representative from the human resources department. This person has considerable clout and can exert leverage on the nurse. He or she can also effectively support and encourage the nurse to accept help. In addition, the authority figure can clearly point out the nurse's options and choices as well as the consequences of any decisions that are made.

In selecting other members of the team, the nurse manager should first draw up a list of all those people in the workplace who have an important relationship with the nurse, either by choice or of necessity. The list should include the names of the following people:

- *Co-workers:* The co-workers named to the list should have a close relationship with the nurse. Co-workers often socialize outside of work and may be aware of problems in a nurse's personal life as well as his professional life. They can offer another perspective and additional information that complements the work-related information the manager has gathered. Co-workers often have a significant impact on the nurse during an intervention because they have worked alongside her and have seen the effects of her addiction firsthand.
- *A recovering nurse:* Including a recovering nurse on the team provides a valuable perspective on the problem. She can truly relate to how the nurse feels and can offer hope, encouragement, and support. It is not essential that the nurse undergoing the intervention know the recovering nurse. Recovering nurses also need not have firsthand knowledge of the nurse's performance problems.
- *Others:* Other possible team members may include nurses, physicians, educators, and individuals who by virtue of their relationship with the nurse have firsthand knowledge of the nurse's problems.

The list may contain 10 or more names. All of these people are prospects for the intervention team, but only a few will actually participate. The best way to narrow the field is to apply a screen. By asking the following 10 questions of themselves, managers can select the best people for the intervention team:

1. If the person were asked to serve on the team, would his or her motive in accepting be to assist the nurse? Interventions are not a time to punish the nurse involved. If the person feels that the nurse should be punished because of his behavior, that person must not be included on the intervention team.
2. Does the person care about the nurse? Intervention team members must be genuinely concerned about the nurse. The atmosphere of the intervention must be one of caring and concern. Anyone who harbors resentments or negative feelings about the nurse will have a negative effect on the intervention. There may even be the question of slander if a team member makes unfounded accusations rather than presenting factual, objective information.

3. Is the person emotionally stable? Team members must be stable because the intervention is an emotional encounter. Very often the nurse being confronted lashes out and verbally attacks those involved in the intervention. Team members must be able to deal with the nurse's reactions without retaliating because they understand the nature of the disease.

4. Does the person have firsthand knowledge of the nurse's inappropriate behaviors or performance? Team members must have firsthand information or else what they say to the nurse will only be hearsay. Exceptions to this guideline are the recovering nurse and the director of nursing or other authority figure who participates in the intervention to apply leverage or to coordinate the meeting.

5. Will the person follow through with the intervention team's plan of action for the chemically dependent nurse? During the intervention, usually the nurse frequently and convincingly denies or minimizes the problem and tries to bargain with the team. Team members must be able to stand firm and not give way to enabling behavior.

   Another common situation is that the nurse agrees to get help but tries to determine where or when. She may promise to see her personal physician later. However, because the physician may not be experienced in chemical dependency treatment, he may actually be enabling the nurse. The team must stand behind its choice of treatment program. The nurse is not in a position to determine the most appropriate evaluation/treatment program.

6. Will the person be able to offer the nurse support in treatment and recovery? Once the intervention is finished and the nurse is in treatment, the nurse will need ongoing support and encouragement that extend into the recovery phase. The nurse very often feels guilty and ashamed of the disease. He needs to know that those who know about his problem support his efforts at finding a solution.

7. Does the person understand the dynamics and nature of chemical dependency? This is a very important question. People selected for the team must at least express a willingness to learn the facts about chemical dependency.

8. Does the person have an untreated problem with alcohol or other drugs? If she does, she may actually sabotage the intervention. A person in recovery, however, could provide an effective role model and reassure and support the nurse.

9. Is the person respected by the nurse? If the information presented during the intervention is to have an impact on the

nurse, the nurse must respect the people on the intervention team or their position.

10. Will the person treat the information and the intervention confidentially? An intervention is very personal and affects the nurse in many ways. It is only proper to treat the information as confidential and not to be discussed with anyone outside the intervention team. Confidentiality also prevents the nurse from finding out that an intervention is planned. If the nurse should find out, he might show up for the meeting. And even if he did show up, his whole denial system would be firmly reinforced before the meeting even started. Either way, the intervention's power would be defused and chances of success would be minimal.

The four or five most qualified people as determined by this screening process should make up the manager's intervention team. The screen should also be applied to the choice of an authority figure to join the team.

Step Three: Identify Financial Resources

During the intervention, the nurse has real concerns about how the proposed evaluation and treatment will be paid for. The team should be prepared to allay those fears so that it can encourage the nurse to seek evaluation and treatment. Therefore, it is important that the nurse manager review the nurse's employee benefits, including medical insurance coverage, leave time, and disability insurance coverage, before the intervention.

The manager should confirm that chemical dependency treatment is covered under the nurse's medical policy. When it is, the next step is to determine the type of treatment covered—inpatient, outpatient, or both. Inpatient treatment can cost anywhere from $10,000 to $30,000 for a 28-day stay. Outpatient treatment costs less, but it may not be appropriate for the nurse involved.

When chemical dependency treatment is not covered under the nurse's medical policy, the manager may need to take up the issue with administration. She may also need to explore alternatives to costly hospital programs, including community-supported programs that offer treatment on a sliding-fee schedule. Many if not most programs supported by public funding have waiting lists for admission to treatment. The most effective way to deal with these issues is to investigate the options available as a matter of establishing a procedure to be followed in all cases, that is, to have identified viable resources for all employees who may need treatment for chemical dependency. The most effective way to address the treatment issue is to establish a hospitalwide policy that provides funding for appropriate treatment for all employees who need it.

Health care facilities may demonstrate real concern for chemically dependent employees and yet fail to pay appropriate attention to the financing of treatment. For example, one employer intervened with a chemically dependent nurse whose health insurance policy did not cover treatment costs. The nurse administrator's concern for the nurse was genuine; however, she believed that if the nurse had really wanted to get well, she would have found the wherewithal to pay for treatment on her own. Obviously, that is not the typical response of health care professionals when someone is having a heart attack, requires treatment for diabetes, or has any other serious medical condition. Health care facilities need to evaluate their policies and procedures, including employee benefits, to determine whether the policies are based on attitudes and judgments that are unfair — and enabling — to chemically dependent employees.

It is also advisable to check how much leave time the nurse has, including annual, disability, and sick leave. A nurse who knows that he has paid leave will be less likely to resist the idea of chemical dependency treatment, and concern over his ability to pay routine bills during treatment will not become a major obstacle. Unfortunately, by the time they reach treatment, chemically dependent nurses often have already used all of their leave time because of addiction-related behavioral and medical problems. In addition, most are experiencing financial difficulties and do not have the financial resources to pay for treatment.

The nurse manager should also find out whether the nurse has a disability policy that would take effect when she entered treatment. Disability coverage helps the nurse avoid the additional stress and anxiety of meeting routine financial obligations (mortgage payments, for example) during treatment; peace of mind on this score makes it much easier for the nurse to concentrate on treatment and recovery.

Step Four: Identify Treatment Programs

In this step, the nurse manager gathers information on available evaluation and treatment programs. Then, he conducts site visits of one or more programs that seem appropriate for the nurse involved. After screening these facilities and seeking out recommendations from people familiar with the programs, the manager chooses the program that promises to best meet the nurse's individual needs. The nurse manager contacts the counselor who would work most closely with the nurse and, if possible, schedules an evaluation.

Finding Potential Treatment Programs

Usually, the nurse manager should focus his search on programs located in the geographic area in which the nurse lives. For outpatient programs especially, the more convenient the location is for the nurse and her family, the more likely the nurse is to enter or agree to treatment in the first place. A facility's geographic location alone, however, should never determine which facility is most appropriate. Many nurses and other people have been effectively treated in locations far from their homes.

Generally, it is advisable to consult several sources of information on treatment programs. Information sources include:

- The state nurses' association peer assistance program or the alternative/diversion program of the state board of nursing
- The state board of nursing or the investigative or disciplinary division in the state
- The facility's employee assistance program
- The local, regional, or state council on alcoholism and drug dependencies
- The local community services directory
- The local or state health department or mental health clinic

When any of these agencies are contacted, the identity of the nurse must be kept confidential unless reporting is required by law.

These sources will probably recommend outpatient as well as inpatient treatment programs. Therefore, it is important that the nurse manager understand how the two types of program differ.

Inpatient programs provide intensive treatment, with therapy groups and activities conducted on a daily basis. Such programs typically last three to four weeks and include a clinically monitored detoxification phase. The nurse resides in the facility for the duration of the program.

Outpatient programs are designed for people who do not require around-the-clock care or who lack the financial resources for inpatient treatment. These programs last anywhere from 4 to 12 weeks, and their content varies considerably. Some are centered on structured, intensive therapeutic activities that last eight hours per day, five days per week. Others conduct three-hour treatment sessions once a week. Each program is structured differently and must be evaluated on its own merits. The choice of outpatient or inpatient treatment is based on the recommendation of the evaluator, not the nurse manager or employer.

The choice of inpatient or outpatient treatment depends on many factors. Unfortunately, it is often dictated by the nurse's health insurance coverage. If the nurse's medical policy covers inpatient treatment and the evaluation indicates that this would be the appropriate treatment, that may be the best option. Usually, by the time a nurse is identified in the workplace as having a potential chemical dependency problem, the disease is fairly advanced, and the nurse probably requires intensive inpatient treatment to ensure the best chances of recovery.

Screening Potential Treatment Programs

As the nurse manager consults various sources, the names of certain treatment programs may come up often. The manager can narrow screening efforts by beginning with those programs. Screening can be done most effectively by visiting treatment facilities to conduct an on-site evaluation. When personal visits are not feasible, the manager can interview program directors and medical directors by phone to narrow the field and visit one or two of the most likely candidates.

The best programs should meet all or most of the following 12 criteria:

1. *The treatment program staff considers chemical dependency a primary disease, not a symptom of some other condition.*
2. *Treatment is delivered by a multidisciplinary team, with a counselor as the primary therapist.* Nurses, physicians, psychologists, allied therapists, clergy, and social workers also serve on the team.
3. *The program follows the 12-step approach pioneered by Alcoholics Anonymous (AA).* Alcoholics Anonymous is a recovery program based on mutual help and adherence to the 12 steps (listed in figure 6-1). Recovering alcoholics in AA meet regularly to share problems, experiences, hope, and strength. The AA approach, which has been adopted by other groups including Narcotics Anonymous and Overeaters Anonymous, has proved to be the most effective in helping alcoholics maintain sobriety.
4. *The treatment program is structured and addresses the physical, mental, emotional, and spiritual needs of its participants.* As already mentioned, chemical dependency affects all areas of a nurse's life; therefore, treatment must address all areas. The treatment method that has proved most effective combines patient

Chapter 6

Figure 6-1. The 12 Steps of Alcoholics Anonymous

1. We admitted we were powerless over alcohol—that our lives had become unmanageable.
2. Came to believe that a Power greater than ourselves could restore us to sanity.
3. Made a decision to turn our will and our lives over to the care of God as we understood Him.
4. Made a searching and fearless moral inventory of ourselves.
5. Admitted to God, to ourselves, and to another human being the exact nature of our wrongs.
6. Were entirely ready to have God remove all these defects of character.
7. Humbly asked Him to remove our shortcomings.
8. Made a list of all the persons we had harmed, and became willing to make amends to them all.
9. Made direct amends to such people wherever possible, except when to do so would injure them or others.
10. Continued to take personal inventory and when we were wrong, promptly admitted it.
11. Sought through prayer and meditation to improve our conscious contact with God as we understood Him, praying only for the knowledge of His will for us and the power to carry that out.
12. Having had a spiritual awakening as the result of these steps, we tried to carry this message to alcoholics and to practice these principles in all our affairs.

Reprinted from *Alcoholics Anonymous*. New York City: Alcoholics Anonymous World Services, Inc., 1976.

education, group therapy, and individual counseling. In addition, comprehensive treatment usually includes adjunct therapies, such as art therapy, music therapy, and recreation therapy (including physical exercise and games).

5. *The treatment staff is experienced in treating the chemically dependent.* The basic professional education that treatment team members received probably did not cover the knowledge and skills required to work successfully with addiction. These skills and knowledge are usually obtained through experience, specific programs of study in addiction treatments, seminars, and continuing education. The nurse manager should ask to see some form of verification that treatment staff members have the necessary experience and education. Certification in addictions treatment is available for most professional groups. The staff should be certified, experienced, or both.

6. *The staff is experienced in treating nurses and other health care professionals.* Although the disease of chemical dependency is the same for all individuals, nurses and other health care professionals have certain characteristics that need to be taken into consideration. These characteristics include a strong need or desire to maintain control, difficulty in assuming the role of patient and allowing others to treat them, extreme guilt and

shame, extremely strong denial, and a strong tendency to intellectualize and become detached from their feelings. Other problems unique to chemically dependent nurses include a concern over licensure issues; the availability of mood-altering drugs in the workplace; rationalization regarding self-medication; and all the beliefs instilled by the nursing culture, such as always putting the patient first (refer to chapter 2).

Chemically dependent nurses have the same disease and treatment needs as any other addicted person. However, because of their unique characteristics and problems, some additional treatment considerations are necessary. Those that cannot be addressed in the core treatment program can often be provided effectively in special group sessions for nurses and other health care professionals. These sessions should be held in addition to — not in place of — the core treatment program.

Nurses and other health care professionals should be treated in the core treatment program alongside other chemically dependent patients. They must not be segregated in their own separate program or living space. Segregation only reinforces their illusion of uniqueness ("We're not like addicts on the street") and strengthens their denial.

7. *The program staff conducts a comprehensive assessment and evaluation of patients upon admission. They then design a treatment plan around each patient's needs.* Assessment and evaluation should include a physical examination and medical history; a history of chemical dependency, including substances used and the effects on family life, personal life, and job/career; a psychological examination and psychological testing; a psychiatric consultation; a social/family assessment; a career/job assessment; an assessment to determine other possible addictions; and an assessment of the patient's understanding of chemical dependency.

Many treatment programs conduct the assessment on an outpatient basis. A staff member trained in assessment interviews the patient and uses specific chemical dependency assessment tools. This preliminary evaluation should not be confused with a comprehensive evaluation. An outpatient assessment usually provides enough information to decide whether the nurse is chemically dependent. A more in-depth evaluation is necessary to make a diagnosis of chemical dependency and arrive at specific recommendations for treatment. The comprehensive evaluation is most often done on an inpatient basis.

8. *The program is accredited by the Joint Commission for Accreditation of Healthcare Organizations and appropriate state agencies, such as the departments of health and mental health.*

9. *The program offers and encourages participation in a family treatment component.* As discussed earlier, chemical dependency is a disease that affects all members of a family, not just the chemically dependent nurse. Typically, family members develop debilitating psychological problems and need to be educated about chemical dependency. They also need to overcome many negative attitudes and learn to discount long-held myths about chemical dependency before their own recovery can begin. A family treatment program helps meet these needs.

10. *An individualized continuing care plan is developed for the nurse prior to discharge.* The plan includes participation in the following: aftercare groups (meetings with other recovering persons to support recovery), often sponsored by the treatment program; individual, group, or family therapy, as needed; self-help groups such as AA, Narcotics Anonymous, and Al-Anon; special nurse support groups sponsored by the treatment program or nurses' associations; and nutrition and exercise programs. Most treatment providers suggest or require that nurses participate in a two-year continuing care program.

11. *The program staff develops a cooperative relationship with, and provides consultation to, the employer.* When the nurse is admitted to the program, the treatment staff contacts the employer about the nurse's job-related problems. The staff also maintains ongoing communication with the employer, especially when the nurse is ready to return to work. For example, the program staff may consult with the employer to determine the most effective time for the nurse to return to work, specific limitations on her nursing practice, the most appropriate work area for the returning nurse, and her job responsibilities. After the nurse returns to work, the employer should consult with program staff in the event any problems arise.

12. *While the nurse is still in treatment, the program staff introduces him to AA, Narcotics Anonymous, groups for recovering professionals, and other appropriate self-help groups.* The staff also requires the nurse to attend meetings of these groups while she is in treatment. The intent is to reinforce the value of the meetings and help the nurse benefit from the experiences of the groups' recovering members.

Treatment programs on the nurse manager's list that best meet these 12 criteria are likely to provide the most comprehensive and effective treatment.

One of these programs may be the hospital's own. If so, should the nurse manager refer the nurse to the hospital's program? Most treatment professionals agree that it is best to treat a nurse in a facility other than the one where she works. This is because the nurse may feel inhibited and unable to overcome fear that "everyone will know about her problems." It is also vitally important that the nurse receive treatment in a setting that is conducive to total honesty and openness. The nurse is likely to feel inhibited in the facility's own program. For these reasons, hospitals and other health care facilities should not treat their own employees in their own chemical dependency programs.

Selecting a Treatment Program

The nurse manager may decide which treatment program to select or consult the intervention team, the hospital's employee assistance program, and/or others on the hospital's staff. Once the choice has been made, it is a good idea to contact the counselor at the treatment program who would serve as the primary therapist for the nurse if he went into treatment. The manager may simply indicate that she believes the nurse may have a problem with alcohol or drugs, as the case may be, and then make an appointment for the nurse to be evaluated. When no date has been set for the intervention, the manager should contact the counselor later, after meeting with the intervention team. At this point, confidentiality should be maintained. It is not necessary to release the nurse's name to the treatment program's staff until the nurse has agreed to evaluation and treatment.

After meeting with the intervention team, the nurse manager may decide to offer the nurse a choice between two evaluation and treatment programs. Freedom to exercise choice in a situation in which she feels that she has no control may help the nurse accept intervention and treatment more readily.

Step Five: Meet with the Intervention Team

The nurse manager meets with other team members once or twice, as necessary, to plan the intervention. During the meetings, the team first reviews key points about the disease of chemical dependency. Then it develops intervention scripts and a plan of action. The team also assigns key roles and tasks to various members, develops a contingency plan, chooses a time and place for the meeting, and rehearses the intervention. These planning steps are explained in detail in the following subsections.

Reviewing Key Facts about Chemical Dependency

The people who have been selected to serve on the intervention team often have various levels of knowledge and expertise in the area of chemical dependency. Therefore, in the early stages of planning, the nurse manager who conducts the intervention should review the key points about chemical dependency with everyone on the team.

The key points to be reviewed include the following:

- Chemical dependency is a treatable disease with definite signs and symptoms. It is not a moral problem or an indication of weak will.
- Chemical dependency is a chronic disease. The nurse is chemically dependent the rest of her life, even when the disease is in remission, a condition that prevails for as long as the individual continues in recovery.
- Because of denial that a problem exists, the nurse is unable to ask for help and initiate treatment. Therefore, help must come from other people.
- Common denial mechanisms that the nurse may use include rationalization, minimization, and projection.
- The nurse has probably been enabled by many people and systems during development and progression of the disease. It is crucial that no further enabling occurs during the intervention.
- There are no quick fixes for the disease of chemical dependency. After intervention, the nurse will require evaluation and treatment before entering a period of recovery, which will be ongoing.

It is especially important to review this information as a team and discuss any concerns or fears the team may have about these points. As necessary, the nurse manager or other designated individual (consultant, treatment counselor, or EAP counselor) should thoroughly explain the psychological terms used to describe the nature of chemical dependency, including *denial, rationalization, minimization, projection,* and *enabling.*

Developing Intervention Scripts

Intervention scripts are written versions of the specific information that each team member will present to the troubled nurse. During the intervention, team members actually read the scripts they have prepared beforehand.

The value of putting this information in writing is that the team members will be able to maintain their objectivity more easily and keep their emotions under better control during the intervention. Team members will also know what to expect from each other during the intervention, and they will tend to feel more comfortable as a result.

Before preparing scripts, team members should share their firsthand information with the team as a whole. Very often, some of the information presented is new to other members and clearly shows the overwhelming problems the nurse has. This verbal recounting usually reinforces each member's commitment to intervene with the nurse.

The next step is to put the verbal accounts in writing. Team members should prepare scripts that are specific, nonjudgmental, objective, and direct. Scripts should also begin on a positive note, with the team members saying how much they care about the nurse, how impressed they were with the nurse's skills and competence in earlier times, and so on.

At this point in intervention planning, it may be helpful for the nurse manager to share some examples of appropriate and inappropriate statements. For example, the following statement is vague and judgmental: "You don't care at all about your appearance." The following revised statement would be more effective: "When you reported for work last Monday, your uniform was wrinkled and had stains on it. Your stockings had runs in them, and you were wearing gray running shoes."

The following statement has the same flaws as the first statement in the preceding example, that is, it is vague and judgmental: "When you called in sick, you were really confused. You sounded out of it." The following revised statement is both objective and factual: "When you called in sick last Monday, I couldn't understand you. Your speech was slurred, your sentences were disjointed, and your excuses didn't make sense."

The following full script for the statement of one team member meets all the criteria for effectiveness:

John, I've worked with you for four years now. During that time, I've come to respect your nursing skills, particularly your wonderful rapport with patients. You have been one of the best nurses on the unit.

Lately, though, I have had some concerns. During the last month you called in sick four times after the shift started. On three days, you did not come in to work or call. Because I was concerned, I called your home but did not get an answer. I didn't know whether you were hurt or in trouble. Something is going on with you and I'm concerned. I care what happens to you, and I want you to get help.

After completing their scripts, team members should read them aloud to each other. This is an opportunity for the team to evaluate the scripts to make sure that they all are as specific, nonjudgmental, objective, and direct as possible. Team members may suggest revisions and improvements.

Writing objective, nonjudgmental scripts is an essential step in preparing for the confrontation with the nurse during the intervention. No one can just show up and confront the nurse with whatever comes to mind at the moment. "Winging it" usually proves costly to the intervention and can undermine its success. The likelihood that derogatory or accusatory statements may slip out is too great. Inappropriate comments can destroy the objective, constructive atmosphere that the team must strive for if the intervention is to meet its goal—getting the nurse to agree to evaluation and treatment.

Agreeing on a Plan of Action

The team must determine what it is going to ask the nurse to do, when it wants her to do it, where it wants her to go, and what the choices are. Typically, the team asks the nurse to undergo an evaluation to rule out chemical dependency. In this way, no one accuses the nurse of being addicted; the team identifies the need to have the issue of chemical dependency addressed. Even when the nurse does admit that she has an alcohol or other drug problem, as some do during the intervention, only an addictions specialist should make the actual diagnosis. The nurse may not be addicted at all but undergoing some psychological trauma instead. Whatever the cause of the nurse's impaired practice, however, some level of treatment is usually indicated.

During the intervention planning meetings, the team also reviews the selection of an evaluation and treatment program. Sometimes the nurse manager may have opted to discuss the various programs available with the team before making a final decision; sometimes he will already have made arrangements with the program staff. Another option is for the team to give the nurse a choice of two or three programs.

The team should also determine when it wants the nurse to undergo evaluation. By the time an intervention takes place, the nurse needs to be evaluated as soon as possible.

Team members usually ask the nurse to get help as part of their scripts. During the intervention, after all the scripts have been read, the nurse manager or the other authority figure on the team urges the nurse to be evaluated specifically for chemical dependency. In the event that the assessment does indicate that chemical dependency is the source of the nurse's work problems, the nurse will already have been informed during the intervention that she will be required to get appropriate treatment.

Before the intervention, the team should agree on what specific directions the nurse manager or other authority figure on the team will give the nurse. Because an intervention is an emotionally draining process, the nurse may experience anger, exhaustion, resentment, relief, confusion, or all of these feelings at the same time. The more directive and specific the team can be, the better.

For example, as part of its plan of action, the team schedules an appointment for the nurse with an addictions specialist. During the intervention, the team informs the nurse that an appointment has been made for him to undergo evaluation and that someone from the team will accompany him to the evaluation and treatment center. It is usually much easier for the nurse to cooperate when relieved of the burden of making decisions. As a result, the evaluation and treatment process can begin immediately.

Assigning Team Roles and Tasks

The team also needs to decide who will play key roles during the intervention and carry out key tasks. Making these decisions beforehand keeps the intervention moving along smoothly, which allows the identified nurse fewer chances to interrupt and object. The following decisions need to be made during the intervention planning meetings:

- *Who will chair the intervention meeting?* The chair is responsible for keeping the process on track. The chair opens the meeting and explains the meeting's purpose to the nurse. The chair sets the tone and maintains control at all times to make sure that team members do not act as enablers and that they stick to the team's plan of action. The person chosen to fill this role must be strong enough to handle any initial resistance and possible verbal attacks from the nurse.
- *Who will go first, second, third, and so forth, when it is time to read the scripts?* The team needs to determine the order of presentation during the planning stage. Such preparation prevents pauses in the flow of the intervention that might give the nurse opportunities to interrupt the presentations and sabotage the intervention.

- *Who will ask the nurse to come to the meeting?* Someone who would usually request a staff meeting should be charged with requesting the nurse to attend. The nurse manager is often the best candidate for this role. Usually, when approaching the nurse, the manager asks her to attend a meeting to discuss recent incidents. The manager should be truthful while at the same time careful not to tip the nurse off to the fact that the meeting is an intervention and that several other people will be there. This has proved to be most effective to prevent arousing the nurse's defense system.
- *Who will make arrangements for the nurse's admission to an evaluation and treatment program?* Because the nurse manager has assessed various programs and met with program staff, she is usually the best person to make the evaluation appointment and the admission arrangements.
- *Who will outline and explain the team's plan of action?* The person who plays this role must be able to exert leverage over the nurse, someone who has enough authority or presence to get the nurse's attention. The nurse manager or another authority figure on the team usually fills this role.
- *Who will ask for the nurse's commitment to the plan?* The team member with the most authority is the best candidate.
- *Who will drive the nurse home after the intervention to pack some belongings and then drive him to the treatment center?* It is important to choose someone who is personally comfortable with the nurse to accompany him, for example, a friend or a recovering nurse who participated in the intervention. Often, the nurse will be very upset, perhaps even distraught, after the intervention. The fear that her job may be in jeopardy is real, and a suicide attempt is a possibility. Therefore, the person who drives the nurse home and to the treatment facility should provide further emotional support. If the nurse is under the influence of alcohol or other drugs at the time of the intervention, it is best to have two people accompany him to the treatment facility. The team should also determine ahead of time who will contact the nurse's family and when that contact will be made. A team member who already knows the family may be the appropriate choice for that task. Otherwise, a hospital administrator or a member of the treatment staff may serve. Very often family members are the nurse's chief enablers, and so deciding when to notify the family about the intervention team's action is a critical concern. If family members are notified before the intervention, they may sabotage the process by informing

the nurse of the planned intervention. Contacting the family after the nurse has agreed to evaluation and/or treatment is usually more effective.

Making Contingency Plans

The team must anticipate the objections the nurse will have to undergoing evaluation and/or treatment and what actions he might take. Preparing its reaction to anticipated contingencies will help the team keep the intervention on course. For example, the following situations sometimes come up during interventions:

- *The nurse angrily stalks out of the room during the intervention.* When this happens, one or preferably two team members should follow her out and ask that she return and at least listen to what the team has to say. Which team members would respond should be decided during the planning meetings.
- *The nurse never shows up for the meeting, or she does show up but walks out early and refuses to return.* When this happens, the intervention team should disband but immediately send a memo requesting the nurse's attendance at another meeting, which should be scheduled as soon as possible. The nurse manager must insist that if the nurse fails to attend the next meeting, disciplinary action will be initiated. The team should decide what disciplinary action is appropriate.
- *The nurse leaves the meeting upset or distraught rather than angry.* One or two team members should follow the nurse out of the room and try to persuade her to return. Failing that, a team member should notify the nurse's spouse, another family member, or a significant other and explain the team's concerns for the nurse. Making a list of the names and phone numbers of these people before the intervention is a wise practice.

  The possibility of the nurse attempting suicide must never be overlooked. The team should be prepared to initiate procedures to admit the nurse involuntarily to a psychiatric facility for his own protection if the nurse demonstrates suicidal behavior or threatens suicide. Because legal procedures for involuntary hospitalization vary from state to state, one of the team members should gather the necessary information from the hospital's social work department, mental health clinic, or employee assistance program before the intervention.
- *The nurse refuses to accept the team's request that she undergo evaluation and treatment.* If this happens, the team should

111

respond by spelling out the consequences of her refusal. The consequences should have been determined during the intervention planning. Often, one of the consequences is termination. (Before the intervention, the nurse manager must have reread the hospital's official policies and procedures on employee termination to make sure that the team's actions are legal and appropriate.)

- *The nurse threatens to sue the team.* The team should be prepared for this reaction, which is a common threat made by people who feel trapped. The nurse may actually carry out his threat, but the lawsuit probably will not go far if the team has solid documentation of the nurse's behaviors and poor performance.
- *The nurse agrees to be evaluated but wants to go at a later date or to someone of her own choosing.* This tactic is often used in an attempt to take control of the intervention. The team should insist that the nurse undergo evaluation immediately or that she cannot resume work before she has undergone evaluation and treatment.
- *The nurse denies that he is an alcoholic or addict.* At this point, the intervention chair needs to make it clear that the team is not accusing the nurse of being an alcoholic or addict but that it is concerned because there is evidence of a real problem. What the team wants is that the nurse get the help needed to solve the problem, whatever it is. When hospital policy requires that all troubled nurses be evaluated for chemical dependency, the policy should be explained to the nurse. However, if the nurse manager has been able to document drug involvement, including diverting hospital drug supplies, he should present that information at the intervention or repeat it if the nurse has already been informed of the information.

Contingency planning improves the effectiveness of the intervention and increases the team's confidence level as well. Team members come to the intervention confident that they are well prepared for the intense emotional encounter to follow.

Setting a Time and Place for the Intervention

As the next-to-last step in planning the intervention, the team schedules the time and place for the intervention. When at all possible, the intervention should be scheduled for a time when the nurse is least likely to be under the influence of mood-altering substances. Also, the intervention should be planned for a day when the evaluation and treatment program staff will be able to see the nurse.

Fridays and the end of the day are not good times for conducting interventions. If the nurse refuses to accept treatment and goes home for the weekend or evening, her denial of the problem will have time to build and become entrenched. Moreover, if the nurse leaves the intervention distraught, she might be suicidal and would have plenty of time alone to carry out her intentions.

The intervention process, including a debriefing for the teams, should be scheduled to last three hours. Often, however, less time is needed. The team should arrive for the intervention 30 or 45 minutes early so that any last-minute questions or concerns can be taken care of. The team members should also forward their calls to someone for the duration of the intervention to avoid being interrupted. It is important that team members feel calm and prepared for the meeting and that last-minute rushing around is avoided.

The room selected for the intervention should be free of interruptions from phone calls and people traffic. The temperature should also be comfortable, and everyone should be seated. In a hospital, it is usually easy to find a conference room or a large office that can meet the team's needs. A phone should be available for making outgoing calls only.

Rehearsing the Intervention

Rehearsing the intervention enhances the team's confidence even more. A rehearsal gives the group a better idea of the sequence of events and how an intervention actually works. During the rehearsal, team members can identify any problems or difficulties they have with the process or their roles. Resolving these issues during rehearsal is preferable to encountering them during the intervention and having to deal with them then.

Typically, the rehearsal is held a day or two before the intervention, with someone recruited to play the nurse on whose behalf the intervention is scheduled. A recovering nurse well established in his or her own recovery makes an ideal candidate. It may also be helpful to view a videotape demonstrating an intervention or to videotape the rehearsal so that it can be critiqued by the team. Training for conducting interventions can be most successful if accomplished in the context of an education/training program carried out before an actual intervention with a specific nurse is planned. (Sources for videotapes are listed in the appendix at the end of this book.)

During the rehearsal, the team should decide where everyone will be seated. The person playing the role of the nurse should be seated next to the team member whose primary function is to support her emotionally during the intervention. The nurse manager usually sits on the nurse's other side, because she will be presenting most of the written information to document behavior and performance problems. This arrangement allows the nurse to easily see the written materials.

Chairs can be arranged in an open circle or around a table. The nurse should not be seated near the door or exit; team members should be seated there instead.

The intervention rehearsal should be conducted just as if it were the real thing, with everyone actively participating and playing their roles. Any snags that develop or questions that arise should be resolved during the rehearsal. Some team members may require a couple of tries before they get their parts down. The rehearsal is the best time to fine-tune preparations. The chair can also invite suggestions for improvements or changes.

Step 6: Conduct the Intervention

By this stage in the process, the team should feel thoroughly prepared and confident that the intervention will be successful. More information on conducting the intervention and a sample intervention, complete with dialogue, are provided in chapter 7.

At the conclusion of the intervention, the team asks the nurse to sign an agreement to undergo evaluation and treatment and a release of information to co-workers. The release of information gives the nurse manager permission to inform co-workers that the nurse has a medical problem, is receiving treatment, and will return to work when appropriate.

Finally, the team holds a debriefing session. For maximum effect, the debriefing should immediately follow the intervention, but often this is not possible because one or two team members are accompanying the nurse to the treatment facility. In such cases, the chair should postpone the debriefing until later in the day when all the team members can be present.

During the debriefing, team members have a chance to vent their feelings and any strong emotions the intervention may have aroused. Team members who may have been verbally abused by the nurse also receive support. The team looks ahead as well, planning how to support the nurse's recovery and return to work. (Chapter 8 discusses the debriefing process and the forms signed by the nurse in detail.)

Summary

An intervention with a chemically dependent nurse has one goal—to get him or her to agree to undergo evaluation and treatment. To achieve that goal, the intervention team presents specific examples of the nurse's inappropriate behavior in a direct, objective, and nonjudgmental way. An intervention is a confrontation but not a personal attack on the nurse. Only the nurse's behavior is the target.

Interventions conducted according to the plan outlined in this chapter typically succeed in getting addicted persons to accept treatment. For the general population, the success rate is 80 percent. Many experts believe the rate is even higher for health care professionals because of their fears about losing their professional status and licensure.

The responsibility for intervening with a chemically dependent nurse lies with the nurse manager who is accountable for the patient care delivered on the unit. The manager is also responsible for providing a safe working environment for all the nursing staff. Too often, the addicted nurse's co-workers take over her duties, and soon their performance, too, is affected. Managers can intervene whenever they see behaviors, attitudes, or actions that are contrary to acceptable nursing practice or inappropriate to the workplace. Once they make the decision to intervene, they need to plan for the event. Key planning tasks include selecting a team to conduct the intervention, identifying financial resources for treatment, and identifying treatment programs. Managers should assess various evaluation and treatment programs well in advance of the intervention, select the best one or two, and make an appointment for the nurse to be evaluated.

In most cases, it is preferable for the manager to meet with the intervention team once or twice before the actual intervention. Team members review key points about the disease of chemical dependency and develop intervention scripts. Reading from prepared scripts helps the intervention to run smoothly and discourages emotional outbursts. The more education the facility employees have received, the better able they are to respond appropriately, especially in a situation requiring an immediate response.

During the planning meetings, the team agrees on a plan of action it will recommend to the nurse, and key roles and tasks related to the intervention are also assigned to team members. A chair for the intervention, usually an authority figure, is chosen.

Contingency planning also helps keep the intervention on course. The team prepares for a number of eventualities. Contingency planning boosts the team's confidence level, and team members arrive for the intervention feeling well prepared.

Just before the actual intervention, the team runs through a rehearsal, with someone (ideally the recovering nurse on the team) assuming the nurse's role. Team members read their scripts and practice their contingency plans to work out any problems or misunderstandings.

Resolving these issues during the rehearsal is preferable to encountering them for the first time during the intervention and having to deal with them on the spot. After all these preparatory steps have been completed, the team is ready for the intervention.

The process outlined in this chapter identifies the nurse manager as the individual who assumes responsibility for a wide range of functions. However, other individuals on staff or outside consultants may facilitate the process of intervention.

□ *References*

1. Morgan, D., and Johnson, V. Intervention: a process for helping impaired physicians. *Journal of the American Medical Association* 69(11):937–39, Nov. 1982.

2. Morgan, D. Intervention. In T. W. Hester, editor. *Professionals and Their Addictions.* Macon, GA: Charter Medical Corporation, 1989.

3. Johnson, V. *Intervention: How to Help Someone Who Doesn't Want Help.* Minneapolis: Johnson Institute, 1986, p. 61.

4. Johnson.

A Sample Intervention

The best way to demonstrate how the key components of an intervention come together is to go through a sample intervention step by step. The intervention described in this chapter demonstrates how careful preparation contributes to the success of the process.

A Troubled Nurse

Janet Tucker is a 43-year-old registered nurse who has been employed at University Hospital for five years. In that time she has held staff positions on both the orthopedic and neurosurgical units. Within the past six months she transferred from the neurosurgical intensive care unit to a general medical–surgical unit. Janet is married and the mother of two children, ages 20 and 16.

Margaret Green is Janet's nurse manager on 7-West, a medical–surgical unit. Over the past three months, she has noticed a decline in Janet's performance and an increase in absenteeism. Also of concern to Margaret has been Janet's attitude. Janet seems to be preoccupied a great deal of the time and very short-tempered with both staff and patients. Complaints from co-workers, patients, and patients' families have increased. Co-workers have reported that they are forced to pick up the slack for Janet because she is not completing her assignments. Very often, they have to run interference among her, the patients, and their families.

In a number of supervisory counseling sessions with Janet concerning her performance, absenteeism, and attitude, Margaret has tried to determine what the underlying problems are and find an appropriate resolution. At each session, Janet has been contrite, saying that financial problems and family responsibilities are taking most of her energy and time. In the past, Margaret allowed Janet to work additional shifts to help with her finances. At times Janet has accused Margaret of being overly critical and responding to staff complaints that she maintains are totally unfounded. Each session concluded with Janet vowing that "things will get better." Still, no substantial changes have occurred, and in fact the situation continues to deteriorate.

During the previous week, Janet called in sick one day. When she reported to work the following day, her appearance was disheveled, her speech hesitant, and she seemed "spaced out." When Margaret confronted her about her appearance, Janet said that she had been up all night, sick. She also retorted, "You're making a big deal out of nothing. With the short staffing, you ought to be glad that I came to work at all."

Margaret told Janet to go home, get some rest, and return the next day at 11 a.m. to meet with her before reporting to duty. Susan McMann, Janet's friend and co-worker, gave her a ride home because the staff was concerned for Janet's safety. Margaret and Susan believed that Janet was under the influence of mood-altering drugs and not able to operate her car safely. While Janet was being driven home, Margaret completed preparations for an intervention to be conducted with Janet at 11 a.m. the next day.

Margaret had identified a pattern of continuing problems that remained unchanged regardless of what she tried to do to correct it. A week and a half earlier, she had approached her supervisor, Lee Jordan, director of medical–surgical nursing, to discuss her concerns about Janet and her conviction that an intervention was necessary. Lee and Margaret began to pull the pieces together and plan a strategy for the intervention at that time.

Documentation of the Problem and Identification of Treatment Resources

Margaret had begun to document Janet's performance and behavior problems a week earlier in preparation for the intervention. She reviewed patient records, controlled drug records, incident reports, attendance and leave records, and Janet's personnel file. There was no doubt in Margaret's mind that Janet's performance had declined, and she was concerned that drugs might have a part in Janet's problems.

Janet's performance evaluations over the past few years indicated a dramatic shift in the quality of her nursing care and concern for her job. Janet had previously received consistent high marks and commendations for her performance. She was recognized for her organizational and technical skills as well as her ability to work well with colleagues, patients, and patients' families. Janet's recent performance evaluations, however, indicated an ongoing though subtle conflict with her supervisor and co-workers. The most recent evaluation was unsatisfactory in many areas, and she did not receive a merit salary increase. In fact, her transfer from the neurological intensive care unit to the medical–surgical unit was suggested by the former nurse manager.

Margaret also discovered that within the past five years since coming to work at University Hospital, Janet had had excused absences for two major surgeries and extensive dental surgery. Janet used her annual leave to supplement her accumulated sick time for the surgeries. Although she had exhausted her leave time, Janet was covered under the hospital's insurance policy for inpatient chemical dependency treatment. She had no disability insurance coverage.

Margaret decided to make tentative arrangements for Janet to enter Chestnut Hill Hospital's chemical dependency treatment program. The hospital had provided similar care to other University Hospital employees in the past and ran an excellent program. Margaret kept Genesis House, which also had an inpatient program, in mind as well, in case Janet wanted an alternative to Chestnut Hill.

The Intervention Team

The incidents of the past week compelled Margaret to take action immediately. The intervention team had already been selected and had met two days earlier to prepare for the intervention. Team members all have firsthand knowledge of how Janet's practice and behavior have been changed. They also have enough authority, leverage, or a special relationship with Janet to have an influence on her during the intervention.

The team includes four members:

- *Lee Jordan*, director of medical–surgical nursing and the intensive care division. She hired Janet five years ago and has come to know her well, because she served as director of the various divisions where Janet worked. Lee is familiar with Janet's past performance and has been pleased with her contributions. She is aware, however, of Janet's current status and problems and is concerned.
- *Margaret Green*, nurse manager of 7-West. Margaret has supervised Janet for the past six months since Janet transferred from the neurosurgical intensive care unit. Before then she had not known Janet, nor was she aware of her job performance. In the past three months, she has noticed problems in Janet's attitude, attendance, and performance. Members of the nursing staff have also approached her with numerous complaints.

119

- *Susan McMann*, Janet's co-worker and friend. Susan has known Janet for five years, ever since she and Janet began working at University Hospital on the orthopedic unit. She currently is working with Janet on 7-West after transferring there four months ago. This is the first time in three years that they have worked together. Susan, who also knows Janet socially, has been concerned about Janet and feels that there is a definite problem. When Susan approached Janet in the past and expressed her concerns, Janet told her that nothing was wrong and to just drop the subject. When nothing seemed to work, Susan approached Margaret to express her concerns.
- *John Taylor*, a physician on University Hospital's medical staff. Janet was an experienced registered nurse when John served as an intern on the orthopedic unit five years ago. Janet helped him through the orthopedic rotation, and they became professional friends. They frequently run into each other at hospital social functions and have always respected each other's professional skills. Dr. Taylor's patients are often assigned to 7-West, and so he frequently sees Janet on the unit. He is concerned about the recent changes in Janet's behavior and performance and has approached both Lee Jordan and Margaret Green to discuss his concerns.

The Intervention Plan

When the team met two days earlier, Margaret shared what she had discovered during her search of past records. Because she believed that drugs were probably at least a part of Janet's problem, she reviewed the key facts about chemical dependency with the team. She urged the team to be especially alert for Janet's attempts to rationalize or minimize problems or to deny in other ways that she had a problem. Team members agreed on a signal that they would use during the intervention if they needed help in dealing with Janet's denial tendencies. The signal would prompt whoever was leading the intervention to jump in and keep everything on track.

Next, Margaret encouraged each team member to share firsthand information on Janet. After doing so, the team proceeded to prepare written scripts for use during the intervention. Margaret emphasized the importance of keeping the scripts factual, objective, and nonjudgmental. As soon as the team members finished writing their scripts, they read them aloud and made revisions based on comments and suggestions from the group.

As the team shared information on Janet, various members became aware of additional problems with her performance and behavior. The severity and extent of Janet's difficulties became even clearer to all of them. It seemed obvious that she had a drug problem. The group felt that they were witnessing her rapid, progressive decline and became committed to getting Janet to accept help.

It did not take the team long to agree on the plan of action it would recommend to Janet. In order for Janet to put her life back in order, they felt she must address her chemical dependency and become and remain sober. Otherwise, the chaos and unmanageability would continue and grow worse. The team would therefore ask Janet to be evaluated for chemical dependency at Chestnut Hill Hospital and to enter treatment immediately. They would offer Genesis House as an alternative if, for some reason, Janet preferred not to go to Chestnut Hill.

After agreeing on a plan of action, the team was ready to assign intervention roles and tasks to various members. It made the following decisions:

- Lee Jordan would chair the intervention. She had been involved in other interventions and knew how to run one effectively.
- The order of script presentation, first to last, would be Margaret Green, Susan McCann, and John Taylor.
- Margaret Green would ask Janet to the meeting. She could best handle this important task without arousing Janet's suspicion because the two have met in the past for supervisory counseling sessions, and the request would not be unusual.
- Margaret Green would also make the necessary arrangements for Janet's admission to Chestnut Hill Hospital.
- Lee Jordan would present the team's plan of action to Janet and gain her commitment to it. Lee is the team member with the most managerial authority, and she has known Janet longer than Margaret has known her.
- Margaret would explain the details of the treatment plan, because she made the arrangements at Chestnut Hill and talked with the staff there.
- Susan McCann, Janet's friend, would drive her home, help her pack, and then drive her to Chestnut Hill. Margaret Green would accompany Susan if it appears that Janet is under the influence of drugs at the time of the intervention.

Lee Jordan brought up the issue of contingency planning. She mentioned that in her first intervention the nurse responded negatively, and because the team had failed to plan for such a reaction members became flustered, and the intervention lost momentum. Because of her past experience, Lee urged the team to take time to plan what it would do in certain situations.

Lee helped the team make the following plans:

- If Janet walked out of the meeting room before or during the intervention, Susan McCann and Margaret Green would follow her out and try to persuade her to return.
- If Janet refused to return or did not show up for the meeting, Margaret Green would send a memo asking her to attend another meeting. Margaret would stress that if Janet did not show up at the next meeting, disciplinary action would be taken that might include termination, as stated in the hospital's policies and procedures.
- If Janet left the room upset or distraught, Susan McCann and Margaret Green would follow her out and assess her emotional status. If she refused to return, Margaret would notify Janet's husband George and express the team's concerns over her emotional health. Margaret would urge George to be at home when Janet arrived there with Susan. As a precaution, Margaret would alert George to the possible need to admit Janet involuntarily to a psychiatric facility for her own protection.
- If Janet refused to undergo evaluation and treatment, Lee Jordan would inform her that she will be terminated unless she reconsiders her decision.
- If Janet threatened to sue, the team would not be intimidated but would proceed with the intervention as planned. As chair, Lee Jordan might acknowledge that Janet has threatened legal action against the team, but the intervention would go on from there.
- If Janet said that she would prefer to see her own physician rather than go to Chestnut Hill, Margaret Green would explain why the team chose Chestnut Hill, emphasizing that University Hospital has been pleased with how Chestnut Hill has cared for its employees in the past. If Janet still expressed reluctance, Margaret would offer Genesis House as an alternative. In any case, Margaret would insist that Janet see an addiction specialist, not her personal physician, for evaluation.
- If Janet denied that she has a drug problem, Lee Jordan would state that the team has documentation that clearly indicates possible drug involvement and remind her that according to hospital policy, evaluation by an addictions specialist is required when drug abuse is a possibility. Lee would reiterate that the team is concerned about her recent behavior and performance and agrees that she should be evaluated for a possible chemical dependency problem. Lee would add that if the evaluation indicated that Janet was not addicted, the team would need to explore other reasons for her declining performance.

With most of the planning tasks completed, Margaret reminded the team that they would hold a rehearsal before the actual intervention. Before adjourning, she called for suggestions on whom they should ask to play Janet's role during the rehearsal. She emphasized that the person should know about chemical dependency and be familiar with the intervention process.

John Taylor suggested Kathy Moore, nurse manager on 4-West, who is a recovering nurse with eight years of sobriety. She had been through her own intervention and knew what it was to be a chemically dependent nurse. She was well regarded throughout the hospital as a competent manager. The rest of the team considered Kathy the perfect choice and directed Margaret to ask Kathy whether she would be available to help with the intervention.

Margaret adjourned the meeting and later that day approached Kathy Moore, who agreed to help.

The Rehearsal

On the morning Janet was sent home from work because of her impaired condition, Margaret called the team together for a rehearsal and notified Kathy Moore. The team met in the conference room that would be used for the intervention. Lee helped Margaret develop a good seating arrangement, which they would also use during the actual intervention. They motioned Kathy, who was playing Janet's role, to a seat near the window and away from the door. Janet's friend Susan McCann sat in the chair on Kathy's right and Margaret sat on Kathy's left. With this arrangement, Janet would be able to see the written records Margaret would refer to during her presentation.

Lee started the intervention rehearsal and explained its purpose to Kathy. As soon as Lee was finished, Margaret began to read her script, followed without pause by Susan and John. At one point, Kathy pretended to leave the room distraught so that the team could implement its contingency plan for that situation. Susan and Margaret followed her out and after five minutes persuaded her to return to the room.

The rehearsal was powerful and had an emotional impact on the entire group, especially Susan, who was visibly upset and close to tears. She had become close friends with Janet over the years, cared about her very much, and was worried about how terrible Janet might feel during the confrontation, as if everyone were ganging up on her.

The team encouraged Susan to talk about her feelings and her concern for Janet. She was worried that Janet might refuse to get help and was convinced that without treatment Janet would continue to get worse and eventually die. Facing this reality was powerful. After much discussion, the team decided that Susan's genuine concern for Janet would definitely have an impact on her and prompt her to get help. The team, including Susan, agreed that she would be able to participate effectively in the intervention without enabling Janet. Susan was an emotionally mature and strong person, a fact that would help her during the intervention. Susan also agreed to take her direction during the intervention from Lee, who would chair the meeting and keep Susan on track.

When the rehearsal was over, the team decided that it should include a recovering nurse in the intervention. They felt that Janet would accept what the team had to say and the action it requested more readily if she had someone to support her. They asked Kathy Moore to serve as an advocate for Janet during the intervention. Kathy had participated in other such interventions and so felt comfortable in that role.

The team left the meeting feeling well prepared to intervene successfully with Janet the next day. They agreed to meet in the nursing conference room between 10:15 and 10:30 a.m. to take care of any last-minute questions or concerns they might have just before the intervention.

The Intervention

Janet reported to Margaret Green's office at 11:10 a.m. the next day. Margaret thanked her for coming and directed her to the conference room for a discussion.

When Janet walked into the conference room, she was surprised to see the team members there. She quickly turned around to look at Margaret. Before she had a chance to say anything, however, Lee Jordan began talking.

Lee: Hello, Janet. I'm glad to see you. Please sit down *(motions to designated chair)*. I believe that you know almost everyone here. Susan McMann and John Taylor. And this is Kathy Moore. Kathy will explain why she is here later on.

   We've asked you here today because we care about you and are concerned about some of the changes we've seen in you recently. This may be difficult for all of us; however, we would like you to listen to what we have to say. Will you do that?

Janet: *(Seems confused and upset; glances at each team member.)* What's this all about? What's going on?

Lee: That's what we want to share with you. Will you listen?

Janet: *(Sits and leans back in the chair with her arms crossed; glares at Lee.)* Well, I'm here now.

Lee: Thank you.

Margaret: Janet, we've known each other about six months now, ever since you came to work on 7-West. You're a good nurse. I've enjoyed working with you and have appreciated your skills, especially with patients who have neurological problems. You have been able to anticipate their concerns and ease their fears.

Lately, I've been concerned about some things that have happened and have worried me. I will share those with you now.

In the last two months you were absent twelve days. On four of those days, you called in at least one hour after the shift had already started. On two other days, you didn't call in at all. I called your home and didn't get an answer. I didn't know whether something had happened to you or not and I was really worried. I didn't hear from you until you reported for duty the next day.

Janet: I already told you I had a family emergency and couldn't call *(sighs)*.

Margaret: *(Does not debate the issue, but continues on with her planned script.)* I have gotten a number of complaints from patients about your care. On Tuesday, Mr. Morrison complained that his pain medication wasn't working. You had charted that he received Demerol® 100 mg at 2:45 p.m. At 3:15 p.m. he was complaining of intense pain and discomfort. The records indicated that he had always reported relief from the medication within 15 minutes of administration. Dr. Taylor happened to be on the unit at the time, and I discussed the situation with him. After we saw Mr. Morrison, I medicated him on Dr. Taylor's orders. Within 15 minutes, Mr. Morrison was relieved and said so. This is not the first time this has happened with one of your patients, and it concerns me.

(Janet shifts position in her chair and looks visibly angry. Her arms are crossed across her chest.)

I did an audit of the controlled drug records for the last two months. I discovered that on six occasions you signed out narcotics for patients who had already left the unit. I also found 10 incidents where you had signed out Demerol® 100 mg for patients receiving Demerol® 75 mg, and the wastages were not co-signed. *(Shows records to Janet.)*

Janet: *(Barely glances at the records.)* No one co-signs those. We're too busy to do that!

Margaret: The hospital's policy states that any wastage of controlled drugs must be witnessed and co-signed.

(Janet's posture becomes more guarded, but she does appear to be listening.)

I am really concerned about your job performance. In the last year, your performance evaluations clearly indicate that you are working below your usual outstanding level. And, at times, your performance has been below acceptable standards. I believe you're familiar with these evaluations? *(Shows Janet the evaluations with Janet's signature.)*

(Janet picks up the evaluations and looks for her signature, which would indicate that she had seen them at the time she was evaluated. When she sees her signature, she pushes them back across the table and leans back in her chair.)

All of this tells me that something is happening with you. I care about you and am concerned.

Susan: *(Begins immediately to share her concerns with Janet so that the process will keep moving and Janet won't have the opportunity to dispute the information and get into a debate.)* Janet, we've been friends a long time now, since we started here five years ago on the ortho unit. You're a terrific nurse. I really value our friendship and have always felt that I could count on you. Lately, though, I've been concerned and worried about you.

Janet: *(Leans forward and glares at Susan.)* Why are you here . . . with them? I thought you were my friend.

Susan: I am your friend. I'm here because I care about you. We always used to talk, but since I came to work on 7-West four months ago, you seem really distant with me. We don't get together for lunch, and at times when I've approached you about going out for coffee after work you've always said no. You seem to be avoiding me. I don't know what's happening.

In the last month, you've called me because you were concerned about missing so much time at work. You asked me to cover for you with Margaret, to tell her that you had gone out of town. When you called me, I could hardly understand you. Your speech was slurred and didn't make sense. When I told you I couldn't lie to Margaret for you, you got really upset. You said that you guessed we really weren't friends anyway and slammed the phone down. I couldn't believe it! I was upset for days.

And yesterday you really scared me. When you came to work, you were 45 minutes late. You looked confused and upset. When I asked you what happened, you said, "Nothing. You're the one with the problem!" Your uniform was wrinkled and stained. That's not like you. You're usually so meticulous about your appearance.

When I took you home yesterday after you saw Margaret, you fell asleep in the car. You were confused when we got to your house. You asked me how you had gotten there. On the way up the stairs, you fell down and cut your knee. It didn't even seem to bother you. After I treated the laceration, I put you to bed and left when you fell asleep and I thought it was safe to go. I called for George to come home and stay with you. When I told him what had happened, he said, "Here we go again." He didn't say anything else. I was afraid to leave you alone, but I needed to get back to work.

Janet: You're overreacting! It was no big deal.

Susan: I was worried all day. When I called you after work, you didn't remember what had happened. You thought I was confused! When I asked about your knee, you didn't know how it had happened.

Janet, I'm really worried. I don't want anything to happen to you, but I'm concerned about the things I've seen. I care about you.

Janet: Yeah. I care about you, too *(sarcastically).*

John: Janet, I asked to be here today because I care about you. When I was an intern on the ortho unit, you helped me get through it. It was a very difficult time for me both professionally and personally. I don't know if I could have gotten through it without your support and encouragement. I could always count on you, and I'll never forget how you helped me. You're a terrific nurse and a wonderful friend.

I'm here because I'm concerned about what I've seen happening to you. Over the last few months, I've had at least four patients complain to me about your care. They've complained that you've been short-tempered with them and have ignored their requests. That's not like you. You're always so responsive to patients and their families.

(Janet is looking at the table and not making eye contact with anyone. She has loosened her crossed arms and seems on the verge of tears.)

Last week I asked you to assist me with a procedure for Mr. Smith. You refused, saying that you didn't see why I needed your help and I'd have to get along without you. I was shocked: That's not like you at all. When I looked for you after I saw Mr. Smith, I couldn't find you anywhere on the unit.

Twice in the last two months, you asked me to prescribe Percodan® for you. You said that you had just undergone dental surgery, were out of medication, and had been unable to get in touch with your dentist. You said that the pain had intensified and you were trying to get to the dentist's as soon as he could see you. I was uncomfortable about it but felt that you must really have needed it or you wouldn't have asked me.

Janet: *(Leans forward in her chair and says sarcastically)* I wouldn't have asked you if I thought it was such an imposition.

John: A few weeks later you asked me again for a prescription to hold you over until you could get to see the oral surgeon. I asked why you still needed the medication and suggested that you see your doctor if you were still having problems. When I said that I could not give you the prescription again, you said that you had never asked me for help before and you would never again. You turned around and walked away. Since that time, whenever I come on the unit, you walk in the other direction and avoid me.

Janet, what's happening? This is not like you. How can I help?

Janet: *(Breaking down)* I don't know how anyone can help.

Lee: Janet, we can help. We're here because we care about you and want to help. With the information everyone has shared with you, it's clear to all of us that your nursing practice has been affected. You are not performing at the level you used to and not at a level that is acceptable for safe nursing care.

Janet: *(Tearfully)* But I'm a good nurse. I care about my patients. I would never do anything to hurt any of them. *(Susan puts her hand on Janet's arm.)*

Lee: *(Leaning toward Janet)* Janet, we know that you're a good nurse and you would never do anything to harm your patients. However, at this time you are having problems that make it difficult for you to practice as you used to. We want to help.

At this time, we want you to get help. We've set up an appointment for you at Chestnut Hill Hospital. You will be admitted for evaluation and then treatment if necessary.

Janet: *(Sits up in her chair and looks directly at Lee.)* Chestnut Hill is for alcoholics and addicts. I'm not an addict!

Lee: We're not saying you're an addict. However, some of the information we have involves drugs. According to hospital policy, we must have the situation evaluated. The problem must first be identified so the appropriate treatment can begin. Things cannot improve without the proper treatment. And you cannot work without getting treatment.

Janet: You mean that you'll fire me if I don't go for treatment?

Lee: Janet, it is not safe for you to practice nursing now. You must get treatment. If you refuse to get treatment, we have no other choice but to let you go. We don't want to do that. We want you to return to University, but if you refuse to get treatment, we have no other choice but to terminate your employment.

Margaret: Janet, I visited Chestnut Hill a few weeks ago to see their program and talk to the staff about the type of services they provide. They will admit you and evaluate your situation and determine what is needed to help you at this time. I spoke with Carrie Galardo, the nurse-counselor, and she is expecting you this afternoon. She will see that you are well taken care of. She will explain the evaluation process to you. We all care about you and want you to get well and come back to University.

(At this time, Margaret does not introduce Genesis House as a choice because Janet has not objected to going to Chestnut Hill. If Janet agrees to go for evaluation/treatment but objects to Chestnut Hill, Genesis House will be offered as an acceptable alternative.)

Janet: I can't go now! They're short-staffed on 7-West. They need me. I'll go next week. I can't afford to go now.

Lee: No, Janet. You need to go now. I appreciate your concern for 7-West, but you need to be cared for now. Your health insurance will pay for any treatment that is necessary. Chestnut Hill is ready to admit you today.

Janet: I just can't do it!

Susan: Janet, I'll go with you. I'll take you home so you can pack a few things to take with you. I'll call George for you. He can meet us at Chestnut Hill. He wants what's best for you.

Janet: But what about my kids? What'll I tell them? They will be so upset!

Susan: Janet, your kids love you. They want you to get well. They will understand. George and I will talk with them. And they will be able to visit with you soon.

Janet: Oh, . . . I just can't . . . I just can't . . . .

Kathy: Janet, I know how difficult this is for you. I understand how you feel. I'm a recovering nurse. I had a problem with alcohol and drugs. A number of years ago, my drinking and drug use caused many problems for me. It affected my nursing practice. I love nursing and my patients, but alcohol and drugs had control of me. The harder I tried to stop, the worse it got. I was doing really bizarre things at work. And my family and my health suffered. I thought that I could handle it by myself, but I couldn't. I was working at another hospital. It got so bad that I was fired. I felt so bad all the time. I didn't know what to do.

(Janet is looking down at her hands. She is wringing a tissue.)

Fortunately, a recovering nurse heard about me and came to see me. She took me to an Alcoholics Anonymous meeting. There, I could really see that there was hope and that I could get help. And that other people cared about me.

(Kathy moves closer to Janet and puts her hand on Janet's arm.)

The next day I went into treatment and my life changed. I learned how to live without alcohol and drugs. It hasn't always been easy, but it's always been better than with alcohol and drugs. It's been eight years, and my life keeps getting better. I still have problems, but I can deal with them now because I'm sober. And I'm back doing the job I love and taking care of patients. I thought that I'd lost all that the day I got fired. But I didn't. I needed to get well.

(Janet is now looking at Kathy and appears to be really listening.)

I've listened to these people today. They care about you very much. They want you to get well. And so do I. I will help you any way that I can. You can call me anytime. I'll be there for you. You need to know that this is not the end of your world but rather the beginning.

I'd like to go with you and Susan. May I?

Janet: I don't know what to do or where to go!

Kathy: Janet. Susan and I will go with you to Chestnut Hill now. OK?

Janet: *(Quietly crying and nodding.)* OK.

The team was relieved and pleased that Janet had accepted help. They hugged her and reinforced her decision and their commitment to support her throughout treatment and recovery.

At the close of the intervention, the team had Janet sign two forms — one agreeing to treatment, the other allowing certain information about her to be disclosed to her co-workers.

In the treatment agreement, Janet essentially agreed to the team's request for evaluation and treatment and allowed the team to share intervention data with the treatment staff. It also reaffirmed the hospital's support for Janet and its desire to retain her as long as she followed the team's plan and returned to safe nursing practice. The release of information form allowed the team to prepare Janet's co-workers for her absence from the unit.

Debriefing for the Intervention Team

Once the intervention was completed and Janet had signed the two forms, the team decided to hold a debriefing session. Because two of its members, Susan and Kathy, were accompanying Janet home, Lee Jordan scheduled the debriefing for late afternoon of the next day.

During the debriefing, team members discussed what went right and what went wrong during the intervention. They concluded that the intervention was successful for several reasons:

- Team members listened to what Janet had to say but did not get entangled in any arguments or debates with her. The emotional level was kept low.
- No one accused Janet overtly of being an addict.
- The team did not insist that she admit or confess anything.
- Because Janet did not object to undergoing evaluation at Chestnut Hill, which was the team's first choice, Genesis House was not brought up. Very often, the nurse being intervened upon is so upset that the only decision he is capable of making is to agree to get help. It is therefore a good idea to suggest one facility and allow the nurse to agree.
- The team stuck to its plan.

The team also discussed their personal feelings and reactions to the intervention and outlined future actions now that Janet had agreed to undergo evaluation and treatment. They spent much of their meeting time planning how they would support Janet's recovery and return to work and exactly what they would say to her co-workers. (The intervention forms and debriefing process are explained in detail in the following chapter.)

Summary

An effective intervention is the key to helping the chemically dependent nurse. Without treatment, the delusional and devastating cycle of chemical dependency will continue. Working as a team to persuade the nurse to agree to evaluation and/or treatment has the greatest potential for success.

In this chapter, the time spent in preparation and the care and concern of the team members created an atmosphere in which the nurse could accept help. The team described in this chapter was exceptionally well prepared and handled all of the nurse's objections and reactions appropriately and compassionately. The value of the intervention rehearsal cannot be overestimated.

Postintervention and Treatment Issues

When the intervention team succeeds in persuading the nurse to undergo evaluation and treatment, the nurse enters a new phase of life. A thorough evaluation is begun upon admission to the treatment facility, and the nurse takes the first important treatment step—detoxification. After detoxification, the nurse participates in individual and group counseling, educational activities, and support groups designed to help her accept the fact that she has a disease, that she must make a lifelong commitment to abstinence from mood-altering drugs, and that she must work to heal all aspects of her life. Upon discharge, she returns to work, enters continuing care, and goes through the early stages of recovery.

Although the intervention team's primary purpose is to persuade the nurse to enter treatment, it also has important tasks to perform at the end of the intervention meeting. These tasks include the following:

- *Completion of various documents:* Intervention documentation helps prevent confusion and disagreements among the nurse, the team, and the employing institution. The documents also create a paper trail in case there are legal challenges later or the employee needs to terminate the nurse for reasons related to her chemical dependency. If the nurse does not comply with all of the agreed-on conditions and further disciplinary action needs to be taken, the intervention documents supply the information needed to support those actions within institutional and legal guidelines. The three documents described in this chapter are the treatment agreement, the intervention report, and the release of information to co-workers.

- *Preparation of plans to support the nurse during and after treatment:* During a debriefing held soon after the intervention, the team also acts to enhance its own support for the nurse. To build support, and with the nurse's permission, the team conducts a meeting with the nurse's co-workers. During the meeting, one or more team members answer questions, allay concerns about the nurse's condition, and generally prepare the nurse's colleagues for his eventual return.
- *Participation in discharge planning and return-to-work planning for the nurse:* These plans are prepared jointly by the treatment team and one or more members of the intervention team (usually the nurse manager or the manager's designee).

This chapter provides practical advice on carrying out each of these tasks. It also contains a brief review of the treatment steps that a chemically dependent nurse goes through. The greater the team's awareness of the nurse's course of treatment, the better able it will be to define its role during treatment. Team members, especially the nurse manager, also gain insights that will prepare them to be effective in their support of the nurse in recovery.

Treatment Agreement and Releases

Once the nurse has agreed to undergo evaluation and treatment for chemical dependency and before she leaves the meeting, the intervention team should ask her to sign a treatment agreement and a release of information to co-workers. The treatment agreement documents the course of action the team and nurse agreed to during the meeting and explains the conditions for a successful return to work. The release of information to co-workers allows the nurse manager to brief co-workers after the nurse has left for treatment. The briefing for co-workers helps stop rumors, builds support for the nurse's return, and continues the process of educating the staff about the problems associated with chemical dependency.

Treatment Agreement

The treatment agreement is an important document that essentially describes the nurse–employer relationship while the nurse is in treatment and recovery. It firmly establishes the nurse's commitment to follow through with the team's request for evaluation and treatment. The agreement also spells out the employer's responsibilities and conditions and documents the nurse's permission to release intervention data to the evaluation and treatment team. Because the agreement is in writing, it also creates a permanent record of events and mutual understandings so that confusion or disagreements are less likely to come up later.

An effective treatment agreement (see figure 8-1 for an example) covers several points, including the following:

- *When and why the intervention meeting was held:* In explaining why the intervention was held, the agreement should focus on job performance issues and behaviors observed in the workplace.
- *What the nurse is specifically agreeing to do:* Typically, the nurse agrees to undergo evaluation and treatment for chemical dependency and to follow the recommendations of the evaluation and treatment team.
- *When and where the nurse will be evaluated and treated:* The time, date, and addictions specialist or treatment center conducting the evaluation should be identified, agreed to by the nurse, and entered into the treatment agreement. Neither the nurse nor the team should leave the intervention meeting without the nurse's commitment to a particular time and place for evaluation. As recommended in chapter 6, the nurse manager should identify one or two effective evaluation and treatment programs before the intervention and, ideally, make an appointment on the nurse's behalf with one or both of them.
- *Conditions under which the nurse will be kept on staff and allowed to return to the workplace:* The Americans with Disabilities Act (ADA) clearly requires employees to "reasonably accommodate" the recovering person who is a "qualified individual with a disability" by giving consideration to the returning employee. Examples of "reasonable accommodation" include job restructuring, part-time work, employee transfer to a vacant position, and other similar actions. One specific area for most recovering nurses is related to the administration of controlled drugs. The workplace must make accommodations for the recovering nurse who cannot administer controlled drugs. This limitation on practice can no longer be used as a reason for disallowing the nurse's return to practice.

    The agreement should reassure the nurse of the employer's support but also spell out the conditions of that support. For example, the agreement usually states that the nurse will be kept on staff with all the benefits to which he is entitled (including vacation and sick leave, medical benefits, insurance coverage,

135

Figure 8-1. Sample Treatment Agreement and Releases

I, _____, an employee of ____(institution's name)____, understand that there are reasonable and legitimate concerns about my job performance. In an effort to address these concerns,

I agree:

(1) To submit to an evaluation for chemical dependency conducted by the provider listed below:

Evaluation/treatment provider: _____ (name)

_____ (address)

_____ (phone)

On ____(specify date)____ At ____(time)____

(2) To sign a release permitting the evaluation and treatment provider to communicate with my employer's representative, _____ (person's name) .

(3) To allow the intervention team, nurse manager, or other designated person to release intervention information to the evaluation and treatment provider.

If the provider determines that I am chemically dependent or have any other illness or condition that interferes with my ability to practice nursing safely or that impairs my judgment,

I agree:

(1) To follow the specific recommendations of the evaluation and treatment team, which can include treatment, continuing care, self-help/mutual-help groups, and other therapies as indicated.

I also understand:

(1) That I will continue to be employed by ____(institution's name)____. I will be assigned to an appropriate position upon my return to work after successfully completing treatment and after being medically cleared to return to work. Although I will continue to be employed by ____(institution's name)____, it may not be possible for me to return to the position I currently hold.

(2) That I will receive any benefits available to me and to which I am entitled at this time while I complete this evaluation and treatment process. These benefits may include annual leave, sick leave, other personal leave, health insurance, disability insurance, and other benefits that may apply.

(3) That when I have been medically cleared to return to the workplace, I will first meet with my supervisor before returning to the job.

(4) That if I fail to adhere to the conditions of this agreement, disciplinary action will be taken, which may include termination of employment with ____(institution's name)____. A report to the state board of nursing will also be filed in compliance with state law.

SIGNED: _____ DATE: _____

WITNESSED: _____ DATE: _____

WITNESSED: _____ DATE: _____

and so on). It also specifies that she will be able to return to the workplace when the treatment team authorizes it, usually after she has successfully completed treatment. In addition, the agreement indicates that the nurse will be placed in a job that will support her recovery and that she may (or may not) return to her former position. This will be determined in conjunction with treatment staff prior to discharge.

The agreement should also spell out the consequences of noncompliance. For example, failure to follow the recommendations of the treatment team would result in disciplinary action, which could include termination. (The institution's policies and procedures must address this issue. See chapter 10 for more information on policies and procedures concerning chemically dependent employees.)

- *When and how reports to the state licensing agency, peer assistance program, or regulatory alternative program will be made:* Some states require that all violations of the Nurse Practice Act involving alcohol, drugs, or impaired practice be reported to the board of nursing or the regulatory alternative program. Other states require that employers report such incidents only if the nurse does not obtain appropriate treatment or does not comply with treatment requirements. Still other states have no mandatory reporting laws at all. Nurse managers should consult with their facility's legal counsel and include the details of any reporting requirements in the treatment agreement.

- *The nurse's agreement to sign a release at the evaluation and treatment center allowing the treatment staff to release information on her evaluation, treatment, and progress to the nurse manager or designated person at the employing institution:* Chemical dependency treatment personnel are prohibited by federal confidentiality laws from releasing information on patients to anyone without specific authorization from those patients. Still, the nurse's employer needs to be informed of the diagnosis and the nurse's progress in treatment in order to make intelligent decisions about job assignments and the nurse's compliance with the treatment agreement. Therefore, the nurse must be instructed and the treatment provider informed that a release signed by the nurse at the time of evaluation and admission is required by the employer.

- *The nurse's permission allowing the nurse manager or other designated person to release intervention data to the evaluation and treatment team:* This information — specifically information on work performance and behaviors observed in the workplace —

is very useful to the evaluator in constructing a complete picture of the nurse. Sharing this information begins the process of collaboration and consultation between the treatment team and the nurse manager–employer throughout treatment, discharge planning, return to work, and continuing care.

• *A treatment agreement covering these points signed and dated by the nurse and witnessed by two other persons:* A copy of the agreement is given to the nurse and the master copy is kept in a confidential file, usually the documentation file.

Release of Information to Co-workers

As mentioned earlier, the chemically dependent nurse does not work in isolation. His co-workers are usually aware of, affected by, and involved in his problems. As a result, the nurse's colleagues have feelings, concerns, and questions that must be addressed. If the questions are not addressed soon after the nurse enters treatment, rumors can run rampant (for example, "She was fired, you know"). Reassuring the nurse's co-workers also helps pave the way for her smooth reentry into the workplace after treatment. The nurse manager or another member of the intervention team, therefore, needs to meet with the nurse's co-workers as soon as possible after the intervention. (Guidelines for conducting the meeting are discussed in detail later in this chapter.)

After the nurse has signed the treatment agreement and before he leaves the intervention meeting, he should be urged to sign a release of information to co-workers. The team should emphasize that it is to the nurse's advantage to have her co-workers understand what has happened. If the nurse refuses to sign a release, it is wise not to force the issue. After the nurse has been in treatment for a while, working with a counselor and making progress, the nurse manager may try again to obtain the release. The treatment counselor and team can be very helpful in presenting the many advantages to the nurse of releasing information to co-workers.

The release of information is a simple form that names someone to conduct the meeting and specifies which co-workers would be informed (see figure 8-2 for an example). Only co-workers with a need to know should be named, such as the colleagues who were most aware of the nurse's problems and the physicians who worked closely with her and expressed concerns about her. Like the treatment agreement, the release should be kept in a secure place, such as the documentation file.

Figure 8-2. Sample Release of Information to Co-workers

I, _____, authorize ___(name of person to conduct meeting)___ to meet with ___(names of individuals or groups of co-workers)___ to inform them of the reason for my absence from the workplace. The purpose of the meeting is to clarify any concerns or questions my co-workers may have.

SIGNED: _____ DATE: _____

WITNESSED: _____ DATE: _____

WITNESSED: _____ DATE: _____

The Intervention Team Debriefing

As soon as possible after the intervention, the team should hold a debriefing. An intervention is an intense experience for everyone involved, not just the nurse. The team focused its time, energy, and hopes on getting the nurse to accept help, and team members often feel emotionally exhausted after the intervention. A debriefing allows the team time to relax, resolve any negative emotions, and discuss improving their intervention skills or learning more effective ways to intervene.

The Timing and Purpose of the Debriefing

The best time to hold a debriefing is immediately after the nurse has left the meeting, when each team member's recollections and reactions are still fresh. When one or more team members are accompanying the nurse to the evaluation and treatment center, the debriefing can be held later, when the entire team is able to reconvene.

A debriefing is a valuable exercise for several reasons:

- It provides team members with the opportunity to express their feelings, concerns, and reactions to the intervention and the nurse.
- It helps the team to clarify and assess what happened during the intervention, focusing on both the actual process as it occurred and the outcome. As team members assess what happened, they review what went right as well as what went wrong.
- It helps the team reaffirm its decision to intervene and reinforces the fact that an intervention was the appropriate action to take, considering the nature and dynamics of chemical dependency.
- It provides support and reassurance for each team member.

- It is the ideal time to discuss how the team will support the nurse during treatment and when he returns to work.

During the debriefing, it is very important to allow and encourage team members to express their feelings about the intervention and the nurse's reactions to it. Team members need to feel that they can freely express their concerns, doubts, emotions, and reactions without fear of being judged or criticized.

Regardless of the intervention's outcome, the team will have reactions, usually both positive and negative, to the experience. Discussing positive emotions during the debriefing reinforces the fact that interventions are an effective, successful method of helping chemically dependent nurses. Discussing negative feelings immediately and receiving support and reassurance helps resolve the emotions. Dealing with negative emotions openly also prevents them from interfering with team members' future support of the nurse's recovery and return to work or their participation on future intervention teams.

Typical negative feelings expressed during intervention debriefings include the following:

- *Guilt:* "Why didn't I do something sooner?" "He has a family to support—he really needs to work." "She accused me of betraying her." Some team members may also feel guilty over what may have felt like "ganging up" on the nurse during the intervention.
- *Anger:* "I can't believe she's blaming us for the problems on the unit." "How could any nurse divert pain medication from her patients?" Although team members have spent considerable time and energy persuading the nurse to accept help in a caring, concerned way, the nurse may have attacked some of them verbally. Unless they have a thorough understanding of chemical dependency or have participated in other interventions, the team members may be angry at the nurse.
- *Doubt:* "Maybe we could have done it some other way." "He has so many problems that I don't see how he's going to get it together."
- *Denial:* "Maybe her drinking's not that bad after all. She really has a lot of problems with her family."

Support, encouragement, and reassurance from fellow team members can usually resolve most negative feelings. If these techniques are not enough, however, the nurse manager or team leader should refer the team member(s) for additional counseling, typically to the employee assistance program (EAP) or an outside counselor. It may also be helpful to have an EAP staff member participate in the debriefing. If an EAP counselor served on the intervention team, he or she could help guide the team through the debriefing process.

As noted earlier, the debriefing is the best time to evaluate how the intervention went. If the process went smoothly, with few unanticipated events, the team can congratulate itself. If the nurse reacted in unanticipated ways that threw the intervention off track, the team needs to analyze what happened. How should the team have responded to keep the intervention on track? Resolving intervention problems during the debriefing improves team members' skills and enables them to learn more effective ways to intervene.

During the debriefing, the team also looks to the future. Specifically, team members discuss how they will support the nurse during treatment and when she returns to the workplace. Common support techniques include the following:

- Sharing intervention information with the evaluation and treatment team
- Planning and conducting an informational meeting with the nurse's co-workers
- Communicating support to the nurse directly through correspondence or phone calls or indirectly through the nurse manager or treatment counselor
- Communicating support for the nurse to his co-workers
- Being direct and positive in interactions with the recovering nurse when she returns to the workplace

The Debriefing Process

The following step-by-step procedure may help guide nurse managers through the debriefing process:

1. During the preparation meetings before for the intervention, the nurse manager should inform the team that a debriefing will be conducted soon after the intervention.
2. After the intervention is finished and the nurse has left for the treatment center, the nurse manager should tell the team members when the debriefing will be held. The nurse manager should notify the team members who left with the nurse of the scheduled meeting time as soon as they return to the hospital.
3. The nurse manager should open the debriefing session by explaining the reasons for the debriefing. He should emphasize

that it allows the team time to relax after an intense confrontation and to evaluate the intervention.

4. The nurse manager should then establish the "rules" that team members will follow during the debriefing. For example:
   - No one will judge another team member's reactions, feelings, or concerns. Everyone is to speak openly without fear of being criticized or judged.
   - No one will put down other team members because of feelings or reactions that they express.
   - Team members will provide support, reassurance, and encouragement to each other during the frank, open discussion.

5. The leader of the team should then ask key questions to encourage team members to talk freely about their feelings and any doubts they may have about the outcome of the process. For example, "I felt angry when Janet blamed me for problems on the unit. Did anyone else feel angry during the intervention? Let's discuss it and deal with it now." The team members should offer support and reassurance to each other as emotions are expressed, acknowledging that nurses often experience real fear during an intervention and lash out at their colleagues as a result. If anyone has difficulty resolving feelings or concerns, the nurse manager should refer him or her to the EAP or an outside counselor.

6. The team should assess the success of the intervention. Did the team achieve its goals? Could things have gone more smoothly? If so, what recommendations would the team make?

7. The team should reaffirm the value of interventions as an effective means of persuading chemically dependent nurses to seek help. If someone on the team has participated in successful interventions before or knows a nurse who was intervened on and later returned to a productive life, this is a good time to share those experiences.

8. The team should plan the informational meeting with the nurse's co-workers to discuss her condition.

9. The team should discuss how it will support the nurse during treatment and when he returns to the workplace.

As with the intervention process itself, it takes practice and experience to conduct a successful debriefing. Nurse managers who feel uncomfortable conducting debriefings can ask an EAP counselor or an outside facilitator to assist with the first few they conduct. As they gain confidence, managers should be able to conduct successful debriefings on their own.

The Intervention Report

Soon after the debriefing or before if the debriefing will take place at a later time, the nurse manager should write an intervention report for the file. This task should be accomplished as soon after the intervention as possible, while the facts and events are still fresh in the manager's mind. The report typically includes the following information:

- The names of the team members
- Specific information on unacceptable job performance and work behaviors that was presented to the nurse
- A description of the nurse's responses (verbal and behavioral)
- The outcome of the intervention
- The agreements and releases that the nurse signed

An intervention report is valuable to the nurse, the intervention team, and the employer for two reasons:

- *It provides information useful to the evaluation and treatment team in determining the nurse's status and treatment needs, a return-to-work plan, and continuing care needs.* Because denial is a major characteristic of the disease of chemical dependency, the evaluation and treatment team must supplement the information supplied by the nurse in order to reach an accurate diagnosis. Most often, chemical dependency is identified by specific signs and symptoms observed by others involved in the nurse's life. Therefore, information in the intervention report on the nurse's workplace problems and behaviors is extremely useful. The nurse manager, EAP counselor, or other designated person usually communicates this information to the treatment team during the evaluation phase.
- *It provides substantial documentation in the event the nurse threatens or attempts to sue the employer for taking disciplinary action against her.* During interventions, nurses may threaten to sue out of fear and denial, a typical reaction of someone who is chemically dependent. By adhering to the intervention plan, responding in an appropriate manner as rehearsed, and preparing a thorough intervention report, nurse managers are usually able to successfully counter such threats.

After completing the intervention report, the nurse manager must keep it in a secure place, such as the confidential documentation file.

The report should be made available only to appropriate staff, usually the manager's supervisor.

The Meeting with Co-workers

Meeting with the nurse's co-workers is critical to the health care facility, the nurse, and the nurse's co-workers for various reasons:

- After the nurse leaves for treatment, rumors circulate. The most common one will be that "she was fired!" This rumor fuels gossip and reinforces the erroneous belief that a nurse found to have a drug or alcohol problem will be fired. This type of thinking only pushes problems underground and makes it more difficult for the health care facility to deal with them. Therefore, rumors must be countered with facts provided by a credible source.
- Co-workers who have worked closely with the nurse usually have numerous questions about his absence from the unit. For example, "What happened?" "Where did he go?" "How can I help him?" These questions need to be answered.
- Co-workers who have actively enabled the nurse in an effort to help her usually feel a sense of failure. They need to understand that, despite their good intentions, the only way the nurse can really be helped is by intervention and subsequent evaluation and treatment by experts.
- At least some co-workers probably have built up very negative feelings toward the nurse. Those who had to fill in when he was absent or late are likely to feel tired, angry, and resentful. Co-workers who frequently bore the brunt of the nurse's mood swings may think, "Good riddance!" They need to be educated about the nature of chemical dependency and come to understand that it is a disease like any other, with disturbing and often disabling symptoms.
- Once co-workers understand the nurse's disease, they may feel that she should leave the nursing profession permanently. They need to realize that although chemical dependency is a chronic disease, it is treatable and that persons in recovery can return to safe nursing practice and a productive work life. They also need to be informed that the health care institution's policies and procedures support the identification, intervention, and retention of troubled employees and that it is illegal to discriminate against disabled employees.

The meeting with co-workers should be held soon after the nurse leaves for evaluation and treatment but only if he signed a release of information to co-workers. The nurse manager and another member of the intervention team should conduct the meeting. If both are inexperienced in running such meetings, an EAP staff member or an experienced outside group facilitator can assist. Since the co-worker group may be quite vocal and present numerous concerns, feelings, and questions that must be dealt with, the group leaders need to go to the meeting prepared to answer any questions.

The following suggestions may prove helpful for managers as they plan and conduct postintervention meetings with co-workers:

- *Describe the exact nature of the meeting and what its goals are.* Major goals usually include informing co-workers of the situation regarding their colleague and allowing them time to express their concerns and feelings about the nurse and her absence.
- *Inform co-workers briefly of what has happened to their colleague.* The nurse manager might say that the nurse was experiencing problems that affected his job performance, that he agreed to undergo evaluation and treatment for chemical dependency, and that he will return to the workplace when appropriate. If the evaluation has not been completed by the time the meeting is conducted, that information should be given to the group. However, no confidential details about the nurse's problems or the intervention should be revealed.

  The nurse's co-workers should also be informed that when the nurse returns to work there may be some limitations on her practice that might affect her ability to administer controlled drugs. Under the Americans with Disabilities Act, co-workers may be required to accept some of the recovering nurse's duties as a "reasonable accommodation" to his disability.

  In addition, the nurse manager should review the institution's policies and procedures for assisting chemically dependent employees and how these were followed in the nurse's case. (Policies and procedures are discussed in depth in chapter 10.)
- *Provide basic information on chemical dependency to help educate the nurse's co-workers.* It should be emphasized that chemical dependency is a chronic but treatable disease with a fairly predictable progression if it is left untreated and that nurses who undergo treatment, abstain from mood-altering drugs, and change the thoughts and behaviors that contributed to their addiction can return to safe nursing practice.

  Any questions that the nurse's co-workers have about the disease should then be answered. If the leader of the meeting cannot answer certain questions, the evaluation and treatment team might be asked to provide answers as long as it does not violate the nurse's right to privacy.

- *Encourage co-workers to express their feelings.* To facilitate a frank, open discussion, the nurse manager could mention some of the common emotions that co-workers feel and ask someone to share her feelings with the group. After one co-worker has opened up, others are likely to follow. The leader of the meeting must maintain a nonjudgmental attitude that encourages the nurse's colleagues to share their real concerns and feelings and allows for resolution.

    Some co-workers may express feelings of powerlessness because they do not know what to do to help. The nurse manager could respond by saying that when the nurse returns to work she will need and welcome her colleagues' support. Until then, co-workers can send cards or letters of support while the nurse is in treatment. This gesture is a very positive one for both co-workers and can mark the beginning of some of the healing for both.

The information meeting with co-workers provides an excellent opportunity to dispel the myth held by most health care professionals that chemical dependency is a moral or character weakness rather than a disease. It is also a forum for educating at least some staff members about the real incidence of chemical dependency and how it can affect them through their contact with chemically dependent patients, colleagues, friends, or relatives. The education provided often enables staff members to identify chemical dependency earlier and assess their own alcohol and drug use.

As part of the educational component of the meeting with the nurse's co-workers, the nurse manager should also briefly explain the process of enabling and provide examples of how a nurse's colleagues may enable the disease. It is essential that co-workers understand the concept of enabling and learn to identify their own enabling behaviors so that they do not resume their enabling habits when the nurse returns to work.

After the meeting with co-workers, the nurse's colleagues will be better able to support her recovery when she returns to work. They will understand what the nurse must do to remain in recovery and why he may have some limitations on practice. They will also expect the nurse to succeed and be less suspicious when she resumes work.

When health care professionals have been properly informed about a nurse's situation and have a chance to work through their feelings toward the nurse, they tend to be more supportive of their colleague while she is in treatment and when she returns to work. This positive outcome occurs most often in facilities that provide ongoing education and training in the disease of chemical dependency for all employees, staff, and management. (Chapter 10 provides more details on a facilitywide educational program.)

Evaluation and Treatment

Members of the intervention team, especially the nurse manager, should have a basic understanding of what transpires during evaluation and treatment for chemical dependency. Every person in treatment takes certain well-defined steps on the road to recovery. Detoxification is perhaps the best known of these steps, but successful treatment deals with much more than the physical impact of the disease and includes the important phase of discharge planning. The rest of this chapter explains the evaluation and treatment process and the nurse manager's crucial role in it.

The Employer–Treatment Team Relationship

It is vital to the nurse's welfare that her employer and the treatment team establish a relationship that fosters sharing needed information and working as a team. The relationship begins when the nurse manager visits or makes phone contact with the treatment facility before the intervention. It continues to unfold as the nurse is evaluated, admitted, treated, and discharged to continuing care.

To help establish a productive relationship, the nurse manager (or someone the manager designates) should convey important information to the evaluation and treatment team and, in turn, request any information that the employer requires. The first step is to notify the evaluation and treatment team that the nurse has agreed to undergo evaluation and treatment as a result of the intervention and that the nurse will arrive at the predetermined time. In addition, the manager should convey the following information:

- The health care facility's requirement that the nurse sign a release of information allowing treatment staff to keep the nurse manager informed of the nurse's progress (an alternative is to have the nurse sign this release during the intervention, after he has agreed to undergo evaluation and treatment)
- That to assist in the evaluation the nurse manager agrees to share with the treatment team any job-related information gathered in preparation for the intervention

- The name of the appropriate person at the health care facility to whom the treatment team should report on the nurse's status in treatment (usually the manager or the employee assistance program representative)
- The frequency of progress reports as required by the facility (weekly reports are usual)
- A request for the name of the primary counselor who will be working with the nurse

This information can be sent or communicated to the treatment facility before the intervention takes place.

If at all possible, the nurse manager or other designated person should visit the treatment center after the nurse has been admitted. A face-to-face meeting with the evaluation and treatment team at this time can be beneficial for all concerned. It helps the nurse manager to develop a relationship with the team that encourages communication throughout the nurse's course of treatment, provides a clearer understanding of the nurse's work-related problems, and assists the team in arriving at a comprehensive and appropriate treatment plan. The nurse will need to sign a release allowing the nurse manager or other designated person to visit the treatment center and discuss the nurse's treatment plan and progress.

The Evaluation Phase

The evaluation and treatment team conducts a comprehensive evaluation of the nurse, including a medical history and physical; a history of alcohol or other drug use; and psychological, psychiatric, and family assessments. Upon completion of the evaluation and on the basis of the information gathered, the team determines whether the nurse is chemically dependent and recommends an appropriate course of treatment. Once the team has reached its decision, it meets with the nurse to discuss its findings and its proposed treatment plan.

The nurse manager should be informed of the team's decision. Usually, by the time the evaluation is complete, the treatment team has been successful in breaking through the nurse's denial and getting her to accept the need for treatment. However, because denial is so strong in chemical dependency, further action may be required to gain the nurse's acceptance. The nurse manager can speed the acceptance process along by calling or meeting with the nurse after the team has informed the nurse of its findings. The manager's input, including a review of the intervention data and the treatment agreement that the nurse signed, can be very beneficial in reinforcing the need for treatment.

If the evaluation reveals that the nurse is not chemically dependent, the evaluation and treatment team should be able to recommend appropriate alternative treatment or evaluation by another qualified professional. If the signs and symptoms observed in the workplace are not attributable to chemical dependency, continued assessment is still necessary. The nurse's problems may be due to mental illness, financial or family problems, professional incompetence, or other conditions. The real cause of the nurse's problems must be identified if chemical dependency is ruled out.

The Treatment Phase

When the evaluation indicates that the nurse is chemically dependent, the first step is primary treatment. This intensive process usually takes place in an inpatient setting and begins the process of recovery. The goals of primary treatment include the following:

- Detoxification
- Overcoming denial
- Commitment to abstinence
- Healing
- Beginning of recovery

A safe, physician-monitored detoxification is the first goal of primary treatment. Because the quantity and variety of drugs used by nurses before entering treatment vary, each nurse must be individually evaluated to arrive at an effective plan for managing withdrawal symptoms. If the nurse is not properly medicated during detoxification, the incidence of untoward reactions—including seizures, tremors, anxiety, and respiratory failure—increases. Without a carefully managed detoxification, the nurse may leave treatment against medical advice in the first few days after admission.

The length of the detoxification phase depends on the type of drug used, the amount used, and the length of time that the nurse has used the drug. Usually, after a few days, the nurse feels well enough to participate in individual and group counseling. During detoxification, the nurse also undergoes a series of evaluations and assessments to determine specific treatment needs.

After the nurse has completed the detoxification phase, the treatment team uses a variety of therapies to achieve the other four goals of primary treatment. Effective treatment helps the chemically dependent nurse to accept that she has a chronic, progressive disease and to understand the nature of chemical dependency. Once the team has

149

broken through the nurse's denial, acceptance comes. Then, the nurse no longer attributes his problems to other people or conditions but accepts the fact that alcohol or other drugs are the cause of his problems and that he has a disease that requires treatment. The nurse also comes to accept the facts that lifelong abstinence is required for ongoing recovery and that she must make a personal commitment to abstain from all mood-altering substances in order to recover from chemical dependency.

Chemical dependency affects the physical, mental, spiritual, and emotional aspects of the nurse's life. During treatment, the nurse must take an intensive look at her life and begin to address the changes that are necessary to maintain sobriety. The process of recovery begins with the nurse changing those behaviors and thoughts that have kept him locked in the despair of chemical dependency. The nurse also learns new, effective, nonchemical ways to deal with reality.

The five goals of primary treatment are achieved through a structured program that includes the following elements:

- Education that is based on group meetings in lecture format that present information on such topics as the 12 steps of addiction recovery, the medical aspects of chemical dependency, the effects of chemical dependency on the family, and the relationship between spirituality and recovery
- Individual and group therapy
- Medical care that includes medically supervised detoxification and medical management of the physical effects of chemical dependency
- Allied therapies such as music, art, and recreation therapy
- Self-help groups such as Alcoholics Anonymous (AA), Narcotics Anonymous (NA), and recovering nurses groups

Completing primary treatment is only the beginning of recovery. The nurse must fulfill her commitment to abstain from all mood-altering chemicals and adhere to the 12-step approach to addiction recovery if she is to maintain long-term sobriety.

Discharge Planning

Studies show that recovering nurses make successful reentries into nursing practice when they have undergone effective intervention and treatment and received strong support in the recovery phase.[1,2] Strong support includes an appropriate plan for discharge, continuing care, and the return to work.

Before the nurse is discharged from primary treatment, the treatment team (with input from the nurse manager) determines the type of follow-up care needed, the nurse's readiness to return to the health care workplace, and the kind of limitations and restrictions that should be imposed on his practice. Usually, by the end of the third week of primary treatment, the treatment team is able to determine whether the nurse can be discharged to continuing care and allowed to return to work or whether intensive extended treatment is needed. The nurse manager needs to consult with the treatment team to decide the proper course of action. When the nurse is to be discharged, the team and manager must map out a return-to-work plan. When the nurse is to enter extended treatment, the manager and team will need to consult again as the nurse nears discharge from extended treatment.

When the nurse is ready to return to nursing practice, the manager's insights into the workplace and the nurse's skills can be invaluable in structuring a continuing care program and return-to-work plan. Together, the treatment team and manager must answer the following questions:

- What limitations or restrictions should be placed on the nurse's practice (for example, area of specialty, responsibilities, and access to controlled drugs)?
- What shifts should the nurse be assigned to?
- How often and with whom should the nurse participate in individual counseling?
- How many times a week should the nurse attend AA, NA, or other meetings of self-help groups?
- How often and where should the nurse attend aftercare or continuing care meetings conducted by the treatment program?
- How often and where should the nurse attend nurse support group meetings?
- How, when, and by whom should the nurse be monitored?

Limitations and Restrictions on Practice

The usual course of action when a recovering nurse returns to practice is to restrict her access to, and responsibility for, administering controlled drugs and any drugs with the potential for abuse or addiction. In general, this restriction applies to all recovering nurses, regardless of their drug of choice. Exceptions to this rule can be made, and a nurse recovering from alcoholism may ask that an exception be made in his case. All such requests should be evaluated by the treatment team. However, most nurses whose drug of choice is alcohol have also used

151

other mood-altering drugs such as Valium®, Xanax®, and Librium® during the active stages of their disease. Alcoholic nurses typically resort to these drugs when alcohol is not available, when it cannot be consumed without discovery, and when medication is needed to relieve the effects of alcohol overdose (hangover).

The restriction on drug access and administration does not mean, however, that the nurse is unstable in recovery or unsafe to practice. It is simply a commonsense support measure for the nurse in early recovery. The nurse needs to experience an established period of sobriety before he again administers mood-altering substances. Some people may have difficulty understanding and accepting this restriction on a nurse, even though they have no problem understanding that an alcoholic bartender should not return to tending bar during the early stages of recovery. Common sense must apply to nurses and other health care workers just as automatically.

Most nurse managers are able to incorporate this restriction into the workplace without any problems. Usually, one of the nurse's co-workers is assigned or volunteers to administer the recovering nurse's medications in exchange for other duties if necessary. When both the recovering nurse and his co-workers are informed of the restriction and understand the rationale, they usually cooperate readily. This effort also complies with the "reasonable accommodation" mandate of the Americans with Disabilities Act. A recovering nurse anxious to prove to everyone that she is again a capable nurse may have difficulty with the restriction at first. If so, the nurse manager can step in as a strong advocate for the nurse's recovery and safe patient care.

In general, the restriction should be in force at least six months, as long as a year, and sometimes longer. Before it is lifted, the nurse should be evaluated by a chemical dependency specialist, usually his continuing care counselor.

The nurse's specialty area of practice also needs to be discussed before she returns to work. Often, the nurse returns to her former unit after treatment. As long as the unit can accommodate the restriction(s) on her practice, it is often the best place for the nurse to begin her recovery.

In some cases, however, assignment to another unit may be the only option. For example, if the nurse manager or the nurse's former co-workers feel very negative about his returning to the unit, he should be reassigned to a unit that is more likely to be supportive, open, and accepting. If the nurse manager on the unit acknowledges that he will find it difficult to supervise the nurse fairly, reassignment to another unit is also indicated for the nurse. Ongoing resentments, suspicions, and negative reactions are detrimental to the nurse's recovery, to her co-workers, and to the unit in general. Ultimately, patient care may be affected. However, when an effective informational meeting for the nurse's co-workers was held earlier, the nurse's colleagues usually respond positively to his return to the unit.

The recovering nurse may also need to be reassigned if her former unit has a high-stress environment. Although all areas of nursing practice entail some stress, the emergency department and trauma units are generally acknowledged to be the most stressful. If the recovering nurse worked on one of these units before entering treatment, he should be assigned to a less stressful unit during the early stages of his recovery.

Frequently, recovering nurses ask to work in the health care facility's chemical dependency treatment program upon their return to practice. The request is understandable, because the nurse's personal experience as a patient has been so self-affirming and positive. However, this is not an appropriate assignment during the first two years after treatment. Nurses assigned to chemical dependency units early in their recovery often relapse and generally find it more difficult to firmly establish their own recovery. Furthermore, patients under treatment for chemical dependency need nurses who are solidly established in their own recovery programs.

Shift Assignment

Shift assignment for the recovering nurse should support his recovery as much as possible. If self-help groups such as AA and NA meet only during early evening hours, the nurse should be assigned a day shift. In some communities, AA and NA groups hold meetings throughout the day, which gives nurse managers more flexibility in shift assignments. The hospital is required under the Americans with Disabilities Act to accommodate the nurse as a recovering drug addict or alcoholic.

Because of the recovering nurse's heavy involvement in support group and aftercare meetings, it is a good idea not to change shift assignments frequently. The relationships she develops within these groups contribute significantly to her recovery; frequent shift changes make it more difficult for her to maintain these relationships and obtain the support she needs.

Another consideration is the level of supervision the nurse receives on various shifts. Because there is more supervision during day shifts and more nurses working at those times, it is usually best to assign a recovering nurse to one of those shifts. The nurse's progress can be more easily monitored and any limitations or restrictions on his practice can be more easily accommodated during day shifts.

Participation in Individual Counseling

Frequently in the treatment phase, problems in the nurse's life are identified that need to be addressed if she is to recover fully. Issues may include family problems, childhood incest, and poor self-esteem. Therefore, the nurse needs to be referred to a counselor or therapist experienced in treating her particular problem. The treatment team should determine how often the nurse should attend individual counseling sessions.

Attendance at Self-Help Group Meetings

Regular, frequent attendance at AA or NA meetings during the nurse's early recovery is essential. Often, the recovering nurse is directed to attend 90 meetings during the first 90 days of recovery in order to firmly establish the recovery phase, as well as build a close connection with the local recovering community, which plays a key role in the nurse's life after treatment.

During treatment or recovery, the nurse is usually urged to find a sponsor within his AA or NA group. The sponsor, who should have a long period of sobriety in recovery, provides close one-on-one support to the nurse. Frequently, nurses and other health care professionals have two sponsors, one who comes from the general community of recovering people and one who is a recovering health care professional. The nurse manager should know who the nurse's sponsors are and how they can be reached at times when additional support is required. Working together, the nurse, the nurse's sponsors, and the nurse manager can often prevent relapses and maintain the nurse's sobriety during stressful times.

Attendance at Aftercare and Continuing Care Meetings

The treatment team will determine how often and where the nurse will be asked to attend aftercare and continuing care meetings. Usually sponsored by the treatment program, the meetings provide the recovering nurse with another opportunity to meet and share common issues and support others who are new to recovery.

Return-to-work agreements may stipulate that a nurse submit verification of attendance at continuing care meetings to his supervisor. In addition to the nurse's actual job performance and behavior in the workplace, the nurse manager can evaluate the nurse's recovery and ability to practice by assessing the nurse's active participation in an ongoing program of recovery, including meetings of this kind.

Attendance at Nurse Support Group Meetings

Groups of recovering nurses (or health care professionals in general) give recovering nurses an opportunity to share issues specifically related to nursing practice and the nurse's role. Often, nurses find it difficult to share their experiences and feelings in a general meeting of people who are consumers of health care services. Nurses fear, and rightly so, that people will become alarmed when they hear about impaired practice, caring for patients while under the influence of drugs or alcohol, and drug diversion. As a consequence, many nurses deal with these issues more openly in peer support groups.

The treatment team should decide where and how often the recovering nurse should attend support group meetings. Nurse support group meetings should be viewed as an important adjunct to, but not a substitute for, AA and NA meetings.

Monitoring Methods and Requirements

Monitoring the recovering nurse after he returns to the workplace is necessary to evaluate his current status in recovery, whether he is abstaining from all mood-altering substances, and whether he is actively working a program of recovery. The treatment team and nurse manager need to discuss the monitoring methods to be used, including reports from treatment providers, drug screens, attendance at recovery meetings, and supervisory evaluations. How often the nurse will be monitored and who will do the monitoring also need to be determined. Usually, if the health care facility has an EAP, an EAP representative can monitor the nurse. Alternatively, an independent chemical dependency specialist can be contracted to monitor the nurse's recovery. If neither of these options exists, someone within nursing administration can monitor all nurses who are recovering from chemical dependency. (More information on monitoring is provided in chapter 10.)

The most effective way to discuss the discharge planning, continuing care, and return-to-work issues is for the nurse manager to plan and attend a conference with the primary counselor at the treatment facility before the nurse is discharged. A face-to-face meeting provides the nurse manager with the best opportunity to clarify and understand what is required for the nurse to achieve a successful recovery. If a face-to-face meeting is not possible, the nurse manager should have a phone conference with the counselor while the nurse is still in treatment. The manager should also ask for a written summary of the discharge plan for the nurse. Once the nurse manager and the treatment team have made all essential decisions and worked out the details, the nurse manager should meet with the nurse before she returns to work. It may be necessary to adjust some of the plan's fine points to accommodate the nurse's preferences.

Summary

Persuading the chemically dependent nurse to agree to evaluation and treatment for chemical dependency is the first step in his eventual recovery and retention. After the intervention, however, the intervention team has several additional tasks to perform to ensure a successful outcome. One of these tasks is to prepare written documents confirming what the team and nurse have agreed on and recounting major facts about the intervention.

Before entering treatment, the nurse should be asked to sign both a treatment agreement and a release of information to co-workers. These documents, along with an intervention report, are filed in a secure place for future reference. If the nurse fails to fulfill her commitment or threatens legal action, these documents supply needed information to support the actions that the health care facility takes.

Demonstrating and building support for the nurse during and after treatment is another important team task. During the team debriefing, held soon after the intervention, team members deal with any negative emotions they may have as a result of confronting the nurse. Clearing away negative feelings paves the way for greater support of the nurse in the days to come. The debriefing also reinforces the team's success. As part of the debriefing, the team also plans how it will demonstrate ongoing support of the nurse and build support among the nurse's co-workers.

Typically, the nurse manager and another member of the intervention team hold a meeting with the nurse's co-workers. At the meeting, they explain briefly why the nurse left for medical treatment, educate co-workers about the disease of chemical dependency, and deal with co-workers' questions and concerns. An educated group of co-workers is far better prepared to support the nurse when he returns to work. The meeting also helps to dispel rumors and raises chemical dependency awareness among staff.

Although the nurse is away from the health care facility during evaluation and treatment, it is essential that her employer and the treatment team share information and work together as a team. When the relationship is a good one, the nurse manager or the manager's designee communicates job-related intervention information to the treatment staff, and the treatment staff shares its findings and decisions (usually limited to diagnosis and course of treatment) with the manager. If the evaluation shows the nurse to be chemically dependent, the nurse manager may also want to meet with the nurse at the treatment center to reinforce the nurse's commitment to follow through with treatment.

As the nurse nears the point of discharge, the nurse manager needs to take an active role in drawing up the discharge and return-to-work plans. Together, the treatment team and manager decide what limitations or restrictions should be imposed on the nurse during early recovery, what shift assignment best meets the nurse's needs, and what individual counseling and support group meetings are necessary to ensure a successful recovery. Because the nurse will be closely monitored during the first few years of recovery, the manager and treatment team will continue to interact long past the discharge date. It is important to remember that in institutions that have EAPs, the responsibilities outlined in this text as those of the nurse manager may be shared with the EAP representative.

☐ *References*

1. Bissell, L., and Haberman, P. W. *Alcoholism in the Professions.* New York City: Oxford University Press, 1984.
2. Hutchinson, S. Chemically dependent nurses: the trajectory toward self-annihilation. *Nursing Research* 35(4):196–201, 1986.

Recovery and Return to Practice

The nurse's return to the workplace where she was employed while in the active stages of chemical dependency is a significant step in the recovery process. Although returning to work represents a positive and reaffirming step for the recovering nurse, this stage may raise concerns among co-workers. The staff members most vested in the nurse's practice and job performance—the nurse manager, co-workers, and even the recovering nurse—often wonder whether he can resume his former duties competently and whether he might return to using drugs or alcohol under the pressure of nursing practice.

This chapter discusses these and other concerns as well as procedures for easing the nurse's return to the workplace, supporting her recovery, and ensuring safe nursing practice. By following the guidelines in this chapter, nurse managers should become more confident about supervising recovering nurses, helping them achieve success on the job, and at the same time ensuring the safety of patients. After learning the typical signs of an impending relapse, managers should also be able to intervene early enough to interrupt the progression to full-blown relapse and resumption of alcohol or drug use.

The Return-to-Work Meeting

The nurse and nurse manager should meet before the nurse returns to the workplace. The primary purpose of the meeting is to review the return-to-work plan developed by the nurse, the nurse manager, and treatment team. Participation in the meeting should be limited to those with a need to know about the nurse's disability to appropriately supervise and support the recovering nurse. The participants typically include the nurse manager, the director of the nursing department, an EAP counselor, an employee relations representative or union representative (if available), and the person assigned to monitor the nurse's progress. (Chapter 10 discusses the criteria for selecting an individual to monitor the recovering nurse when he returns to the workplace.)

The meeting should be held in a place that provides privacy and freedom from interruptions and distractions. The atmosphere during the meeting should be one of openness and concern. It is best to define the agenda for the meeting on the basis of specific goals. The following list suggests the most important goals of any return-to-work meeting:

1. To discuss the concerns of the nurse manager and the recovering nurse regarding her return to the workplace
2. To respond to any of the recovering nurse's concerns or questions related to reentry issues, including:
   - Unit assignment, shift assignment, and limitations on practice: Under the Americans with Disabilities Act, reasonable accommodation for the nurse's disability is required. The nurse manager should be prepared to answer all of the nurse's questions. Decisions on unit assignment, shift assignment, and limitations on practice should already have been made during discharge planning meetings.
   - Job performance evaluation procedures:
     - The specific forms to be used in evaluating the nurse's job performance should be discussed. The most effective approach is to use the same evaluation tools that the health care facility employs with all nurses.
     - The frequency of evaluations should be agreed upon. A recovering nurse should be evaluated as often as necessary to benefit the nurse and to provide the manager with feedback about the nurse's performance. A useful guideline is to conduct evaluations one month, three months, and six months after the nurse returns to the workplace and subsequently to follow the institution's usual performance evaluation schedule. If the early evaluations are less than favorable, steps must be taken to correct or improve the situation. Consultation with the EAP staff, the nurse's treatment and continuing care counselor, or another appropriate resource is recommended.
     - The person who will evaluate the nurse should be determined. The nurse must know who will be evaluating her. (Usually, it is the nurse manager.)
3. To review the continuing care plan and the treatment team's recommendations: The treatment team should have provided

the nurse manager with a written summary of its recommendations for the nurse's continuing care. The specific plan becomes part of the return-to-work agreement (described in detail later in this chapter) and includes attendance at and participation in AA or NA meetings, nurse support group meetings (or meetings of other health care professional support groups), continuing care meetings (usually held at the treatment center), and individual counseling if required.

4. To review the process that will be used to monitor the nurse's recovery: The recovering nurse is monitored in order to verify that he is continuing in recovery and can safely practice nursing. (Specific monitoring procedures are described in chapter 10.) The information gathered during the monitoring process also can protect the nurse from false accusations. Monitoring methods may include alcohol or other drug screenings; written reports from counselors, supervisors, and sponsors; self-reports; and verification of attendance at AA or NA and other support group meetings.

5. To assess the nurse's readiness to return to the job as well as her understanding of the recovery process: The assessment can be done through open discussion and by the nurse's responses to the manager's questions and comments. A discussion of assessment techniques with the nurse's treatment counselor before the meeting can help prepare the manager.

6. To finalize the return-to-work agreement: The agreement covers the conditions for continuing employment and the consequences of noncompliance. (An example of the agreement is provided later in this chapter.)

When the nurse manager follows the agenda outlined above and conveys an expectation of success, the return-to-work meeting can prove instrumental in the nurse's recovery and smooth reentry into the workplace.

Dealing with the Manager's Concerns

Typically, the nurse manager has a number of concerns that need to be discussed with the nurse at the return-to-work meeting. It is perfectly normal to have some questions or doubts about the nurse's ability to return to the workplace. Directly discussing concerns with others, including the recovering nurse, is the manager's most effective tool for resolving these issues.

Before the return-to-work meeting, the nurse manager may find it helpful to discuss specific concerns with the nurse's continuing care counselor, other treatment personnel, the institution's EAP staff, or the manager's supervisor (if he or she is experienced in this area). Concerns that require direct input from the nurse should be discussed frankly during the meeting. Because chemical dependency treatment programs emphasize the need for honesty in all interactions, the recovering nurse should be prepared to honestly and directly discuss issues surrounding her recovery and any questions the manager may have. When the manager and the recovering nurse address these matters openly, a level of communication will be established that sets an important standard for future communications and support during recovery. Frank and open discussion like this also helps to prevent nurse managers from enabling recovering nurses.

The most common questions that nurse managers have when recovering nurses return to practice include these:

- *Will the nurse be able to do the job without creating problems?* The nurse manager does not want to see a resumption of the performance problems that led to the intervention and subsequent treatment. The manager should review those problems with the nurse and ask him to explain how the situation has changed and why those problems will not recur.
- *Can treatment really work?* In the past, the nurse manager probably made a number of attempts to help the nurse and failed. The manager may wonder, "How is this time any different?" To find out whether the nurse's thinking has changed, the manager could specifically ask, "What can you tell me about your treatment and recovery?" When the nurse acknowledges that she is an alcoholic or an addict, it indicates an acceptance of her disease and the ongoing program of recovery. The nurse should also articulate specific information about what she needs to do in order to maintain sobriety: attending AA or NA, nurse support group, and continuing care meetings; having a sponsor; abstaining from all mood-altering chemicals; and making sobriety the number-one priority in her life.
- *What is my role? What is my relationship with the nurse now?* Very often, nurse managers erroneously think that they are supposed to act as counselors to the recovering nurse. The manager's role should be the same as it always has been. The nurse has a professional continuing care counselor and other identified resources that she can turn to for counseling and guidance on recovery issues. What the nurse needs from his manager is support and assistance in doing a good job and recognition when he does his job well. The most effective ways in which the nurse

manager can support the nurse's recovery include verbally communicating support; conveying a positive attitude; assigning a realistic schedule; being flexible in allowing her to attend support meetings; providing immediate attention and suggestions regarding her performance, attitude, and behavior when they are below professional standards; recognizing and praising appropriate performance; and refusing to act as an enabler.

To establish the nurse's recovery on a firm foundation, the manager may want to ask the nurse additional questions during the return-to-work meeting. The following questions focus on issues of importance to both the nurse and the manager:

- *How do you plan to respond to questions or concerns that co-workers express about your return?* The nurse should realize that co-workers will have questions and concerns that need to be addressed immediately in an honest and open manner. This question should prompt her to prepare for dealing with her colleagues if she has not already done so. The nurse may request the manager's support in approaching and talking with staff.
- *What stressors did you experience in your job before going into treatment? What do you consider to be the stressors as you return now? How will you handle this stress?* The nurse should be able to explain past and present stressors and describe how she will handle stress now without using alcohol or other drugs.
- *How can I best support your return and recovery?* The nurse may identify specific areas, including flexibility in scheduling to accommodate his need to attend continuing care meetings; no requests for overtime; no floating to other units; feedback on job performance; a general feeling of support; immediate confrontation when the manager becomes concerned about performance issues; and additional training or orientation to job responsibilities if the nurse is assuming a new job or if he is feeling uncertain of his skill levels.

Because the nurse manager is responsible for the delivery of safe, competent patient care, she needs to feel comfortable with the recovering nurse and confident in the care she will provide. The nurse's responses throughout the meeting should indicate an acceptance of her disease and a willingness to do whatever it takes to maintain sobriety. The manager should look for an open and honest manner. The nurse may show some anxiety, but this is normal because she wants to do well and show that she can resume safe, competent nursing practice.

The nurse should also demonstrate an understanding that his behavior during the active phase of chemical dependency adversely affected his co-workers.

Accommodating the Nurse's Concerns

The recovering nurse also has concerns and fears about returning to the workplace that need to be dealt with during the return-to-work meeting. For instance, the nurse will probably be concerned about how he will handle being around drugs, how he will cope with stress in the workplace, how others will respond to his return, how he will prove that he can do the job well, and how he will balance his job responsibilities with ongoing treatment and continuing care meetings.

For the preceding few weeks, the recovering nurse underwent treatment in an environment that was responsive to her specific needs and goals. Now, she is returning to an environment where her last interaction was negative and she left many people, both supervisors and co-workers, with negative feelings and pessimism about her ability to recover. Some of the nurse's immediate questions as he returns to the workplace will probably include the following:

- *Can I still do the job?* The nurse last practiced while under the influence of alcohol or other drugs. She will be concerned about her ability to meet professional nursing standards. The nurse manager should assure her that she is a competent nurse, that some anxiety is normal, and that the manager will be there to support her and provide any needed assistance.
- *How will others respond to me? Will they accept my return? Will they forgive me? Will they ever trust me again?* It is normal for the nurse to feel anxious about facing his co-workers after chemical dependency treatment. During treatment, she has become acutely aware of her past performance and behavior problems and how they affected her co-workers. The nurse manager should let the nurse know of his co-workers' concerns as well as their support.

    If the nurse's co-workers had an opportunity to discuss their concerns and reactions when the nurse left the workplace to enter treatment, they are likely to be more supportive of the returning nurse. If they have specific questions concerning the nurse's treatment and recovery, they should be encouraged to ask the nurse directly. The resulting dialogue can often be a healing experience for everyone involved. The recovering nurse has an opportunity to make amends and the co-workers have an opportunity to offer support.

- *How will I handle the pressure and stress of work without alcohol or other drugs?* While in treatment the recovering nurse learned new ways of dealing with stress. However, she will feel some natural anxiety upon returning to the workplace. The nurse manager may anticipate the nurse's fears by reinforcing the fact that she has the manager's support and that she will be successful.

   For example, the manager and nurse might discuss a situation that the nurse had difficulty handling in the past, before treatment. The nurse could be encouraged to discuss his feelings and choose effective strategies to handle the situation.

   During recovery, the nurse will try very hard to be perfect, to prove to herself and her co-workers that she is capable of doing the work. Frequently, however, the recovering nurse may impose unrealistic expectations on herself.

- *How will the patients react to me? Will they know that I'm a recovering alcoholic or addict?* The nurse manager should assure the nurse that patients will not be informed of the nurse's history and current status as a recovering alcoholic or addict. There usually is no reason for patients to be so informed. Due to continuing misunderstandings regarding chemical dependency, sharing this information with most patients serves no useful purpose and may unduly alarm them.

   There are some exceptions to this guideline, however. At times, nurses have shared their status as a recovering person with patients and families and doing so has proved beneficial to everyone. One situation involved a recovering narcotic addict who was about to undergo surgery and was understandably anxious about receiving narcotic analgesics after surgery. He was concerned about a relapse. The nurse was able to allay some anxiety by informing the patient that she was also recovering. She discussed his concerns with the attending surgeon, who was not experienced in treating recovering addicts and had dismissed the patient's concerns, which significantly added to the patient's stress and anxiety. As a result of the nurse's intervention with the patient and the surgeon, an appropriate postsurgical analgesic treatment plan was developed with the patient's input that addressed his concerns, reduced his presurgical anxiety, and facilitated an uneventful recovery. Also key to the patient's successful recovery was the entire nursing staff's understanding of his particular concerns and needs, which was due in part to the ongoing education provided by the facility.

Open and honest discussion of these and any other questions and anxieties that the nurse has prior to resuming work will pave the way for a smooth transition for everyone.

Working Out a Return-to-Work Agreement

During the return-to-work meeting, the recovering nurse should be asked to sign an agreement that clearly outlines the employer's expectations and the nurse's responsibilities. A copy of the agreement should be given to the nurse, and the original placed in the confidential intervention documentation file.

When the nurse began employment with the health care facility, she was considered competent, qualified, and able to perform her duties unencumbered. Therefore, she was evaluated according to the usual policies and procedures of the institution. Now that he has been identified as having a disease that affects his ability to practice nursing safely, the facility must monitor his recovery to ensure safe, uncompromised, nonimpaired nursing practice. The return-to-work agreement governs this monitoring period.

In essence, the agreement establishes ground rules for the new relationship between the recovering nurse and her employer. The following points should be included in the agreement:

- A statement by the nurse recognizing that he is chemically dependent
- The nurse's agreement to several conditions:
  - To remain abstinent from all mood-altering substances, including over-the-counter medicines
  - To retain a primary physician experienced in treating recovering alcoholics or addicts (any prescription drugs that the nurse uses must be authorized by this physician)
  - To participate in the continuing care program recommended by the treatment team for the specified period of time
  - To submit to random drug screening as requested
  - To comply with state peer assistance or alternative/diversion program requirements if the state maintains such a program
  - To abide by the terms of the agreement for the specified period of time
- A statement of the consequences if the nurse fails to comply with the agreement

A sample return-to-work agreement is shown in figure 9-1. The nurse manager should use and adapt it as necessary. (Because state laws

Figure 9-1. Sample Return-to-Work Agreement

I, _____, recognize that I am recovering from the disease of chemical dependency and wish to continue my recovery. I agree to the following conditions:

1. To completely abstain from the use of alcohol, marijuana, cocaine, stimulants, narcotics, sedatives, tranquilizers, and all other mood-altering, mind-altering, and potentially addictive drugs or substances, prescribed or otherwise. This includes over-the-counter medications containing any of the above or other mood-altering substances.

2. To obtain the services of a physician for my medical care who is an addictions specialist or recognized as being knowledgeable in the treatment of recovering alcoholics and addicts. If I am unable to locate a specialist in my area, I shall inform my personal physician, _____, of the conditions of this agreement and request that he or she not prescribe any of the above substances for me unless there is no reasonable medical alternative. Before prescribing any of the above substances, my physician will consult with the physician who was responsible for my medical care while I was being treated for chemical dependency. If, after the consultation, any narcotics, sedatives, tranquilizers, or other mood-altering or mind-altering or potentially addictive drugs are determined to be necessary, my physician shall immediately notify my supervisor, _____, in writing. I give permission for my personal physician to release the information to my supervisor and authorize my supervisor to contact my personal physician in matters concerning my health and recovery.

3. To inform my supervisor in writing of the physician responsible for my medical care at the time of this agreement. If I need to obtain a physician, I will do so within one week of signing this agreement and will notify my supervisor in writing.

4. To request a referral from my primary physician if the services of any other physicians are necessary. My primary physician can therefore brief them on my special needs. I shall also inform other physicians of my history of chemical dependency and of the terms of this agreement.

5. To inform my spouse or significant other person, _____, of the conditions of this agreement, giving him or her permission to contact my supervisor if there is ever any concern about my use of alcohol or other drugs or about my behavior. I give permission to my supervisor to contact the person named above.
(Work phone) _____ (Home phone) _____

6. To participate in the continuing care program as recommended by my treatment counselor for the recommended period of time, _____. I understand that regular attendance is required. I will submit signed attendance sheets indicating my compliance with this agreement.

7. To participate in and attend approved support group meetings on the following schedule:

    AA/NA: _____ times per week

    Others as required:

    1. _____: _____ times per week
       (type of meeting)
    2. _____: _____ times per week
       (type of meeting)

(Continued on next page)

Figure 9-1. (Continued)

I further agree to provide signed weekly attendance reports to my supervisor or the person monitoring my recovery. I understand that regular attendance is required. I understand that I must obtain a sponsor through my AA or NA group and supply my supervisor with his or her name within a week of returning to work.

8. To submit to random drug screenings when requested by my supervisor or other appropriate employee. I shall inform whoever requests the screenings of any substance or medication, prescribed or otherwise, that I have taken prior to submitting a specimen for analysis.

9. (Insert if applicable to your employee's situation.) To comply with the conditions/requirements of the ___(name of peer assistance or alternative program)___

10. To abide by the terms of this agreement for a period of _____, or until I have satisfactorily complied with them.

11. If I, _____, do not comply with the above terms of this agreement, I understand that disciplinary action will be taken, which may include termination from employment.

12. I understand that nothing in this agreement is intended to supersede (name of institution's) policies and procedures concerning its employees. I further understand that my employment may be terminated at any time by (name of institution) in accordance with policies and procedures in effect at the time of termination.

_____   _____
Employee's Signature   Date

_____   _____
Supervisor/Manager's Signature   Date

_____   _____
Administrator/CEO's Signature   Date

differ, the agreement should also be reviewed by the facility's legal counsel.) Employers and recovering nurses have found that spelling out expectations in a written agreement of this kind is extremely helpful. The agreement provides the structure necessary to ensure that nurses receive strong and consistent support during recovery. When return-to-work agreements are adhered to, they can prevent enabling of the nurse and reinforce the goals of recovery.

Supervision of the Recovering Nurse

Nurse managers are often unsure of how to treat the nurse once she returns to the unit and resumes most of her duties. Some managers may become overprotective, others hypercritical. In general, managers should manage and supervise the nurse in the same way they did in the past but provide an extra degree of support. The following suggestions for the nurse manager have proved effective in supervising recovering nurses:

- *Be yourself.* The nurse manager is not the nurse's counselor or confessor, but the nurse's supervisor does play an important role in her recovery and in the quality of patient care. The manager should follow effective management and supervisory procedures as he has done in the past.
- *Expect success.* Verbalizing support and confidence in the recovering nurse's ability to do well will have a powerful impact. The manager needs to be positive in outlook, and she can be when she understands the nature of chemical dependency and communicates often and openly with the nurse and the treatment team or counselor.
- *Be clear about expectations.* The recovering nurse should have a clear understanding of how he is expected to perform and behave when he returns to practice. This understanding can be achieved through the return-to-work agreement and a review of the nurse's job description as well as the facility's performance evaluation procedures.
- *Communicate openly with the nurse.* The nurse manager must not delay in confronting the nurse if problems begin to surface. Successful recovery depends on honesty, and communications with the nurse must be direct. If at any time the manager has questions about the nurse's ability to perform the job, the manager should be open and ask questions. Behavior, attitude, or performance problems should be dealt with immediately. They may signal the beginning of a relapse or lead to a relapse if unchecked. (Relapses are discussed later in this chapter.) The nurse manager must not enable or try to protect the nurse or ignore situations that would be addressed if other nurses were involved. Delay only allows the problem to continue and worsen, with potentially harmful consequences for the nurse, staff, and patients.

  If the manager observes the nurse acting short-tempered with a patient, discovers that the nurse has not attended support group meetings, or notes a pattern of tardiness or absence from the nursing unit, the manager should discuss the problem with the nurse as soon as possible. As during the intervention, the manager should present objective information about his observations and concerns. After confronting the nurse directly, the manager should follow up by discussing the situation with the person monitoring the nurse's recovery or the nurse's counselor. It is always best for the manager to discuss potential problems with others who are also actively involved and concerned with the nurse's recovery. The behavior or situation the manager observed may be a one-time occurrence or a reaction to immediate stress. On the other hand, the manager's observations may corroborate concerns that the nurse's monitor or counselor has about the nurse's progress in recovery.

- *Be fair and consistent in the standards applied to the nurse.* The nurse should be held responsible for meeting the standards required of all employees. She must not be expected to perform better than other nurses to prove that she is again competent and safe to practice.
- *Tap available resources as needed to help you support the nurse's recovery.* Whenever the nurse manager has questions or concerns about the nurse's behavior, attitude, or job performance, she should contact the health care facility's EAP staff (if available), the nurse's counselor, or the state peer assistance or alternative program (if available). These individuals and groups can help the manager understand the dynamics of recovery, identify any potential problem areas, and intervene appropriately.
- *Direct all questions to the recovering nurse.* When the nurse returns to the workplace, all questions regarding his recovery, treatment, and the like should be directed to the nurse for response. If the nurse manager conducted an informational meeting for the nurse's co-workers when the nurse left for treatment and if the hospital maintains an ongoing educational program on chemical dependency for all staff, the nurse's co-workers should be able to resume working alongside the nurse and address their concerns or questions to the nurse directly.

Often, after returning to work, the recovering nurse requests a meeting with her co-workers to answer any questions. She uses this time to explain her disease and what she learned in treatment, as well as to express gratitude for the staff's concern and caring attitude. Frequently, the staff members are already aware of the nurse's restriction on administering controlled drugs and will even offer suggestions on how to implement it. Such meetings can be very effective in establishing a positive tone and open atmosphere.

By following these guidelines, the manager can establish a strong, supportive relationship with the nurse and, at the same time, fulfill her responsibilities for ensuring competent patient care.

Coordination with the Nurse's New Manager

As part of the discharge plan for the recovering nurse, the nurse's manager and treatment team may decide that she should resume work on a different unit. Their decision may be based on the stress level of the unit she worked on previously or on other factors. When this is the case, the new nurse manager needs to be briefed. Staff members on the new unit may also have questions that should be addressed. If the institution has a program to effectively educate all employees about chemical dependency in the workplace and to prepare all nurse managers for supervising recovering nurses, the reentry process will be much less difficult for recovering nurses, supervisors, and co-workers.

Regardless of whether the facility has such a program, the recovering nurse's previous supervisor should brief the new manager on the nurse's particular situation. The new manager should receive information about the recovering nurse's treatment; the dynamics of chemical dependency (if the health care facility has not educated staff on the subject); how the nurse's performance has been affected; the conditions of reemployment as spelled out in the return-to-work agreement; and any limitations or restrictions on the nurse's practice.

The manager who will supervise the returning nurse must also be involved in the return-to-work meeting. During the meeting, the new manager should feel free to voice any concerns she has about the recovering nurse and how the nurse will function on the unit. This meeting can help set a positive tone for the new working relationship. The new manager should also receive a copy of the return-to-work agreement.

Nurses on the unit may or may not be aware of the nurse's chemical dependency and recent treatment. If they are not, it is not the responsibility of the new manager (nor is it appropriate) to discuss the nurse's case with staff. If the nurse has limitations on his practice that will require coverage by other staff members, the manager should inform only those who will perform various functions for the recovering nurse. Moreover, the information shared should be specific to the task. If staff members ask questions or have concerns of a more personal nature or questions pertaining to the nurse's treatment, they should be directed to the recovering nurse.

The new nurse manager and the recovering nurse should discuss how the recovering nurse wants to deal with co-workers' questions. This topic can be addressed most effectively at the return-to-work meeting. Many nurses opt to meet with their new co-workers when they start on the unit. They explain their recent treatment experience and how it will affect their practice. If the health care facility conducts ongoing chemical dependency education programs for all employees and the issue of chemical dependency and recovering staff members is an open, accepted topic, recovering nurses will not be an anomaly.

Staff on the nurse's new unit should not be expected, nor asked, to "watch the nurse closely." The proper mode of operations should be that all inappropriate behaviors and procedures, regardless of whether they are demonstrated by the recovering nurse or others, are reported to the nurse manager. To specifically earmark the recovering nurse only causes added suspicion and increases stress on the unit. Through an effective facilitywide program, all staff can be educated to identify inappropriate behaviors and practices and made aware of the necessary policies and procedures to follow.

Signs of Relapse

Like patients with chronic diseases such as diabetes and heart disease, nurses recovering from chemical dependency can experience a relapse. A relapse is basically a recurrence of disease symptoms after a period of improvement.

For the alcoholic or addict, a relapse does not start with the resumption of drinking or other drug use. It begins as a progression of behavioral and cognitive patterns that reactivate feelings of isolation, denial, elevated stress, and impaired judgment.[1] These are the same patterns that were present when the individual was actively drinking or using other drugs. Most recovering alcoholics and addicts refer to these patterns as "stinkin' thinkin'." The patterns usually set the stage for a resumption of drug or alcohol use.

As part of the treatment program, the nurse and his family were briefed on the warning signs of relapse. Such information improves the chances that someone would intervene if warning signs appeared and thereby prevent the nurse's slide into full-blown relapse.

The nurse's manager also needs to understand the dynamics of relapse. The manager is in the best position to intervene when the early signs of relapse start manifesting themselves in the workplace.

A 1973 study identified the typical warning signs of relapse among alcoholics.[2] The same signs are generally accepted as applying to those addicted to other drugs as well. Using these warning signs, Gorski and Miller developed an 11-stage model of the progression toward relapse. By recognizing these stages nurse managers can intervene early and interrupt the progression:

1. *Stressful change.* The progression toward relapse begins with changes in the individual's life that trigger stress and changes

in thinking and attitude, which, in turn, bring about behavioral changes that interfere with ongoing recovery. Very often as a result, the recovering person develops a negative attitude toward the recovery program and feels that he need not follow the recommended practices.

Because of the potential for relapse in early recovery, nurses are urged to refrain from making changes in their lives that might alter their daily structure, increase their stress levels, and weaken their commitment to working for recovery. Specific changes that individuals should delay making in early recovery include moving, changing jobs, getting married or divorced, changing careers, making major purchases or sales, accumulating sizable debts, and scheduling elective surgery. There are exceptions to these general guidelines based on the need to make certain changes in order to progress in recovery. Among valid exceptions are separation or divorce if the nurse is in danger and changing jobs if the nurse is unable to return to the same job because it is detrimental to her recovery or she has been fired.

2. *Elevated stress:* The second stage is characterized by an elevated stress level. Recovering alcoholics and addicts have a low tolerance for stress during the early stages of recovery. Changes in their lives often produce stress, which in turn causes them to overreact. They may then resort to negative methods for coping with the added stress, including the use of mood-altering substances.

3. *Resumption of denial thinking:* With increased stress, the recovering nurse tends to deny the presence of the stress. She may also start denying other problems in her life. In this way, the denial mechanisms that characterized the active stages of her disease are reactivated.

4. *Postacute withdrawal:* In addition to experiencing withdrawal symptoms during treatment, a nurse may undergo withdrawal symptoms later as a result of elevated stress. Even though the nurse may still be abstaining from alcohol or other drugs, he can develop problems in cognitive and emotional processes and suffer memory lapses typical of withdrawal. The nurse may make inappropriate decisions and poor judgments; display mood swings and emotional outbursts; blame others for circumstances and events; become defensive, isolated, and suspicious of others; and become unable to recall events or remember responsibilities.

5. *Behavioral changes:* With the progression of denial, chronic elevated stress, impaired cognitive and emotional processes, and

173

memory problems, the recovering nurse's behavior changes. Her actions may become inappropriate, for example, she may become abusive or irrational.

6. *Social breakdown:* The nurse's interactions with family, friends, and co-workers deteriorate because of his behavioral changes. Family and friends avoid the nurse in order to prevent problems. Those who were previously supportive withdraw as a way of coping with the changes.

7. *Loss of structure in daily life:* The nurse's life soon becomes chaotic and unmanageable. She may abandon her recovery program and change habits or daily routines. Her ability to attend to personal needs such as eating, attending support group meetings, and exercising is lost. Unless someone intervenes, she continues a downward spiral toward active chemical dependency.

8. *Loss of judgment:* As the recovering nurse's life loses structure and his social relationships deteriorate, he becomes confused and cannot solve problems or make decisions. A characteristic during this phase is the absence of balance in many life areas. For example, the nurse may become emotionally numb or overreact to everyday situations.

9. *Loss of control:* The nurse eventually loses control of her thought processes and behaviors. She can no longer make rational choices and loses any ability to halt the downward slide into relapse. The only way she can get well is if others intervene.

10. *Option reduction:* The alcoholic or addict believes that he is unable to interrupt the downward slide, that he is no longer in control, and that there are very few alternatives. Only negative consequences seem likely—insanity, physical or emotional collapse, suicide, or resumption of alcohol or other drug use.

11. *Acute degeneration:* In the final stage, the nurse resumes drinking or using drugs, develops emotional or stress-related illnesses, or attempts suicide.

As this 11-stage model shows, the relapse process often begins long before the recovering nurse resumes drinking or using drugs. How much time it takes for the nurse to progress to a resumption of drinking or drug use varies considerably. Some recovering addicts and alcoholics start using again at various points in the 11-stage model. Therefore, the earlier the nurse manager identifies the symptoms of relapse, the sooner the progression to actual use can be interrupted and the nurse returned to active recovery.

If the nurse manager observes any signs or symptoms that indicate a possible problem, she should refer the nurse to the facility's EAP counselor or the nurse's continuing care counselor. If there is specific information to confirm that the nurse is using mood-altering substances, has violated or failed to adhere to the return-to-work agreement, or has exhibited unacceptable job behavior, the nurse should be immediately removed from practice. The next step is to have her recovery status and ability to practice nursing evaluated by a chemical dependency specialist. The specialist may be an EAP counselor, the nurse's continuing care counselor, or some other outside chemical dependency specialist. Once the evaluation is complete, the specialist's recommendations should be implemented before the nurse returns to work. The institution's policies and procedures must also address the consequences of relapse. (See chapter 10 for more information.)

Summary

The nurse's return to the workplace marks a significant step in recovery. To pave the way for a successful return and to ensure a continuing high level of patient care, the nurse manager should meet with the nurse to discuss various issues before the nurse returns to work. During the return-to-work meeting, they review the nurse's shift assignments, any practice limitations, procedures for evaluating job performance, and the nurse's continuing care plan. The manager also briefs the nurse on how the health care facility plans to monitor her progress in recovery. A return-to-work agreement, which the nurse is asked to sign, governs the new relationship between the nurse and his employer. It stipulates the conditions for continued employment and the consequences of noncompliance.

The return-to-work meeting should also set the stage for open, frank communication between manager and nurse in the coming months. Toward that end, the manager and nurse need to deal openly with their concerns as the nurse prepares to resume most of her duties.

Once the nurse resumes practice, the manager should apply the same high nursing standards to him as to other nurses on the unit. Being overly protective will not help the nurse achieve success. When problems arise, they need to be discussed and resolved promptly. Neither should the manager be overly critical. The best approach is to expect the nurse to succeed and follow the same effective management and supervisory procedures as always.

If the nurse returns to a unit other than her former one, an informational meeting with new co-workers may help allay fears and concerns. The new manager should also participate in a return-to-work meeting with the nurse and freely express any concerns.

Because chemical dependency is a chronic disease, recovering nurses sometimes suffer relapses. Before the resumption of drinking or using drugs, however, a nurse headed for relapse most often displays identifiable cognitive and behavioral symptoms reminiscent of active chemical dependency. Researchers have described 11 stages in the progression toward relapse. When managers are familiar with these stages, they will be better able to interrupt the progression and help the nurse return to active recovery.

☐ *References*

1. Gorski, T. T., and Miller, M. *Counseling for Relapse Prevention.* Independence, MO: Herald House – Independence Press, 1982.
2. Gorski and Miller.

A Facilitywide Alcohol and Drug Program

To implement the process outlined in this book, nurse managers need the support of their institutions' administrators. The institution can most effectively facilitate the successful management of chemically dependent nurses by establishing a facilitywide alcohol and drug program that includes comprehensive policies and procedures and ongoing education for all staff.

The nurse manager can take a number of action steps to enlist the administration's support for, and endorsement of, such a program:

- She can become educated about chemical dependency and impaired practice issues, including the nature of the disease, its signs and symptoms, intervention techniques, and reentry to the workplace—in short, all the topics covered in this book.
- He can actively solicit support from his peers for a program that advocates a drug-free workplace.
- She can explain the benefits of such a program to the administration. Major benefits include the retention of qualified, experienced staff; decreased liability; improved staff morale; and enhanced patient safety.
- He can explain (with the advice of legal counsel) the requirements of the Americans with Disabilities Act (ADA) and the extent to which the legislation affects the facility's human resources policies and procedures.
- She can emphasize that the American Hospital Association encourages health care institutions to develop substance abuse policies and procedures and supports the identification, treatment, and rehabilitation of chemically dependent employees.

- He can volunteer his time to help establish the program and participate on the task force that will draw up policies and procedures.

The American Hospital Association's Board of Trustees recently adopted a general policy strongly encouraging health care institutions to adopt written substance abuse policies, including provisions for drug and alcohol testing. The AHA policy supports the premise that establishing drug-testing programs will result in improved patient and employee safety, improved quality of care, a healthier work force, heightened employee efficiency, and an improved community image. The policy also states that without appropriate employee education, treatment, and rehabilitation, the benefits of implementing a testing policy cannot be fully realized.

This chapter presents information and guidelines to help health care facilities develop a comprehensive alcohol and drug program that encourages consistent management of chemically dependent employees.

Policies and Procedures

Clearly defined policies and procedures for the management of chemically dependent employees provide for consistent responses to situations that affect the safety of patients and staff, as well as the overall operations of the health care facility. Without clear, effective policies and procedures, the problems caused by alcohol or other drug use among employees are usually ignored or inappropriately handled, chemically dependent employees are enabled, and the quality of patient care is compromised.

To guide the development of effective policies and procedures, the facility should first establish the institution's philosophy on chemical dependency in the workplace. This philosophy reflects the beliefs, attitudes, and general values of the institution with respect to the use of mood-altering chemicals in the health care environment. It also reaffirms the facility's responsibility for providing a safe environment that promotes the health and welfare of both patients and employees. The philosophy statement becomes the basis for the policies and procedures document.

A strong statement of philosophy (an example is shown in figure 10-1) contains at least these essential concepts:

- The use of alcohol or other drugs (in fact, all mood-altering chemicals) in the workplace is unacceptable.

Figure 10-1. Policies and Procedures Governing Employees' Use of Alcohol or Other Drugs in the Workplace

Philosophy

__(Name of hospital)__ recognizes that we have a responsibility to provide high-quality, safe patient care that is uncompromised by employees' use of mood-altering substances. We also have a responsibility to our employees to provide them with a drug-free environment that promotes their health and welfare. The use of alcohol or other drugs (all mood-altering chemicals) in the workplace is therefore unacceptable (except in specific, individual cases when they are legitimately prescribed by a physician and their use has been approved by this institution's employee health physician).

We recognize that chemical dependency is a disease that affects all levels of employees and impairs their job performance, placing them, their co-workers, and patients at risk. The security of this institution and the productivity of our employees, as well as the public's confidence and trust in us, are adversely affected by the incidence of use of mood-altering chemicals by employees.

We believe that chemical dependency is a disease that can be effectively treated and that recovering employees can return to their former level of uncompromised, high-quality job performance. As an employer, we are responsible for providing our employees with the education and resources necessary to encourage them to receive appropriate treatment. We are also responsible for encouraging employees to return to their jobs when patient care and the employees' own recovery will not be adversely affected.

This philosophy is implemented through the following fitness-for-duty policy.

Fitness-for-Duty Policy

General Statement

To provide a safe environment and to promote the health and welfare of its patients, visitors, and employees, the hospital will require its employees to report for work and perform their duties free of illegal drugs, alcohol, and other drugs that may impair job performance. For purposes of this policy, illegal drugs shall be defined as any drug or controlled substance, the use of which is illegal under either state or federal law without a prescription. Illegal drugs include, but are not limited to, those controlled substances listed in __(name of state statute)__ .

To enforce this policy, the hospital will test employees for drugs upon reasonable suspicion of drug and alcohol use, as a condition of employment.

Objective

It is the intent of this policy to maintain a drug-free work force and to assist employees in remedying any medical problems related to the use of drugs, including alcohol.

Supervisor's Responsibilities

"Fitness for duty" in a hospital requires that employees be free from the effects of illegal drugs or alcohol. Supervisors are therefore responsible for:

1. Observing the behavior of employees on the job so as to prevent those who are unfit for duty from working in the hospital.
2. Making a determination of fitness for duty based on their knowledge and training and on the training being provided to them by this institution. Supervisors are not expected to diagnose the cause of the employee's unfit behavior.
3. Attempting to get another supervisor to verify his or her observations of an employee's unfit behavior.
4. Notifying the department head whenever an employee is removed from duty for reasons of being unfit.

Employee's Responsibilities

Every employee is responsible for:

1. Being fit for duty when reporting to work.

(Continued on next page)

Figure 10-1. (Continued)

2. Reporting to his or her supervisor behavior that raises a doubt as to the fitness for work of a fellow employee.

Policy

The following practices are to be considered conditions of hospital employment and should be consistently adhered to:

1. Employees are required to notify their immediate supervisor (or the supervisor-in-charge) when reporting for duty or in the course of their work shifts whenever their use of any prescribed or other drug may adversely affect their ability to satisfactorily perform normal job duties.
2. Employees must comply with a fitness-for-duty evaluation, which includes an intervention and may include urine or blood testing for chemical levels (such as alcohol, illegal drugs, and other drugs) when directed to do so by their immediate supervisor (or the supervisor-in-charge) and the department director. The evaluation may occur when an employee reports for duty or during the course of his or her shift.
3. Supervisors should comply with this document's fitness-for-duty evaluation procedures (see later section) whenever they request an evaluation. It is especially important for them to document their observations that the employee is unable to initiate or continue normal work duties due to unfitness for duty.
4. Employees should follow the hospital's rules of conduct, which are, by their nature, conditions of employment. The following on-the-job behaviors are considered inappropriate forms of conduct:
   a. Using, possessing, or selling any alcoholic beverages or illegal drugs on hospital premises, including the hospital parking lot.
   b. Reporting to work with illegal drugs in their body or under the influence of alcohol, even though they may not show any adverse outward effects from doing so.
   c. Reporting for work or continuing to work in a condition unfit for duty or failing to follow the hospital's fitness-for-duty policy and procedures.

Confidentiality

The results of a fitness-for-duty evaluation will be kept in a medical record maintained by the employee health service. Under no circumstances will the record or the results contained therein be released to any party (except hospital supervisory or management employees on a need-to-know basis) without the employee's prior written permission unless the hospital is required to do so pursuant to legal or administrative complaint procedures.

Procedure for Fitness-for-Duty Evaluation

The supervisor should assume the following responsibilities:

1. Document observed deficiencies in employee performance or behavior. Documentation must be directly related to the employee's inability to satisfactorily perform his or her job due to the possible adverse influence of alcohol or illegal drug usage. Observed deficiencies may include, but are not limited to, the following:
   a. Drowsiness and/or sleepiness
   b. Odor of alcohol on breath
   c. Slurred or incoherent speech
   d. Unusually aggressive behavior
   e. Unexplained work errors
   f. Unexplained changes in mood
   g. Lack of manual dexterity
   h. Lack of coordination
   i. Unexplained work-related accidents or injuries
2. Attempt to get another supervisor to verify observations.
3. Arrange a meeting (intervention) with the employee. Contact the resource person responsible for conducting interventions. If time permits, the supervisor or the resource person should

Figure 10-1. (Continued)

assemble an intervention team. There may not be enough time, however, if the nurse's condition poses an immediate danger to patients.

During Weekday Hours (8:00 a.m.–5:00 p.m)

1. The supervisor notifies department head of need for evaluation.
2. The department head and supervisor discuss concerns with employee and request an evaluation, including an intervention.
3. Drug testing may be requested and performed if the employee appears to be impaired because of alcohol or other drug use. The employee should be tested if there is a reasonable suspicion that he or she has used alcohol or drugs. For purposes of this policy, "reasonable suspicion" shall be defined as suspicion supported by circumstances sufficiently strong to warrant a cautious person to believe, based on specific objective facts and rational inferences drawn from them, that the employee has been using alcohol or illegal drugs.
4. Intervention is set with   (identify resource person and phone number) . Time permitting, a team of co-workers shall participate in the intervention.
5. The employee is transported safely to the facility where assessment for chemical dependency will be performed. If the assessment is scheduled for the following day, the employee is safely transported home.
6. The person conducting the assessment will notify the department head of his or her findings, along with a recommendation as to whether the employee is able to return to work immediately or requires treatment.
7. The employee shall be paid for the time required for an assessment and may use accrued leave for treatment.
8. If the employee refuses to be assessed and undergo treatment, as recommended, disciplinary action will be taken, including possible termination.
9. If the employee receives treatment and returns to work, he or she will be expected to follow return-to-work guidelines, as outlined by the supervisor, department head, and EAP counselor.

During Evenings and Nights (5:00 p.m.–8:00 a.m.) and Weekends

1. The supervisor notifies the department head of the need for evaluation.
2. The supervisor and department head discuss their concerns with the employee.
3. Drug testing may be requested and performed if there is a reasonable suspicion that the employee is under the influence of alcohol or other drugs.
4. If the unfitness for duty appears to be due to illness, the employee's recent medical history should be reviewed with the employee health service.
5. Assist the employee in getting home safely.
6. Schedule an intervention for the following workday (contact the resource person).
7. The employee is transported safely to the facility where the assessment for chemical dependency will be performed. If the assessment will not take place until the next day, the employee is safely transported home if he or she is still under the influence of drugs or alcohol.
8. The person conducting the assessment will notify the department head of his or her findings, along with a recommendation as to whether the employee can return to work immediately or requires treatment.
9. The employee shall be paid for the time required to undergo an assessment and may use accrued leave for treatment.
10. If the employee refuses to be assessed and undergo treatment as recommended, disciplinary action will be taken, including possible termination.
11. If the employee receives treatment and returns to work, he or she will be expected to follow return-to-work guidelines as outlined by the supervisor, department head, and EAP counselor.

- Chemical dependency is a disease that affects all levels of employees; impairs job performance; and places affected employees, their co-workers, and patients at risk.
- Chemical dependency adversely affects:
  - the health and safety of patients and staff.
  - the security and productivity of the institution.
  - the public's confidence and trust.
- The institution is responsible for providing a safe environment that promotes the health and welfare of its staff and patients.
- The disease of chemical dependency can be effectively treated, and recovering employees can return to an acceptable, unimpaired level of job performance.
- The institution has a responsibility to provide appropriate intervention and treatment services for affected employees. The institution also has a responsibility to permit recovering employees to return to their jobs when their work will be consistent with patient safety and the facility's standards of care.

To develop a philosophy statement, as well as related policies and procedures, the facility should select an interdisciplinary task force of 8 to 12 employees. Task force members can be chosen by the administrator or someone acting on his or her behalf, usually the vice-president of human resources or the director of personnel. The task force should reflect all major personnel groups in the facility to ensure that the policies and procedures developed will be appropriate, responsive to various needs, and widely accepted. Groups typically represented on the task force include nursing, labor relations, unions, legal affairs, medicine, security, human resources/personnel, and employee assistance.

If the facility does not maintain an employee assistance program (EAP), it is advisable to call in an outside chemical dependency consultant to act as an adviser for the task force. The consultant selected should not only be experienced in the field of addictions, but also knowledgeable in managerial issues. The facility's philosophy statement, policies, and procedures need to reflect the most current information available in the chemical dependency field.

Fitness-for-Duty Policy

Once the philosophy statement has been drawn up and received the administration's approval, the task force is ready to work on the rest of the policy and procedure document. The document, usually known as a fitness-for-duty policy, covers a number of issues. The issues are usually discussed and debated by the task force before they are committed to written form once a consensus has been reached.

Issues that should be covered in any fitness-for-duty policy include the following:

- *The facility's rationale, or objective, in developing the policy:* A goal suggested by the National Institute on Drug Abuse is "to maintain a work force that is free from impairment by alcohol/other drug effects detrimental to productivity, safety, and health, and at the same time to offer any employee who does not meet those conditions an opportunity, consistent with other employee policies, to be restored to an optimal level of performance."[1]
- *The facility's expectations regarding drug use in the workplace:* Examples include these: the use of illegal drugs and mood-altering chemicals, including alcohol, will be prohibited; the use of any drugs except over-the-counter medications must be through legal prescription.
- *Action(s) the facility will take:* When an employee is found to be using prohibited drugs, the facility may require referral for assessment and evaluation, treatment for the presenting condition, and disciplinary action.
- *The ways in which the facility will demonstrate its support for treatment:* Support for treatment is manifested in the benefits offered by the facility to affected employees, including health insurance coverage for treatment; sick leaves, personal leaves, and leaves of absence for treatment; and disability coverage. The facility's support is also manifested by its commitment to retain recovering employees on staff when to do so is consistent with patient safety.
- *The ways in which the facility will demonstrate its support for recovering employees:* Examples include these: employees may return to former or comparable positions as recovery permits; every effort will be made to return employees to the positions they held before treatment as long as they can perform job responsibilities within limitations or restrictions. The ADA requires reasonable accommodations for recovering chemically dependent employees.
- *The facility's requirement that the policies and procedures will be strictly adhered to and closely monitored to ensure that they are administered fairly and consistently.*
- *The facility's requirement that all referrals, whether self-referrals or supervisory referrals, will be accorded maximum respect for employee confidentiality, consistent with safety and security*

issues: Information gathered on an employee's use of alcohol or other drugs, including results of drug tests and documentation of impaired job performance, will be kept in a separate supervisory file, not in the employee's official personnel file. Information regarding the employee's admission to treatment will be shared with his or her co-workers only with the employee's knowledge and permission.

- *The follow-up procedures the facility will execute when alcohol or other drug use in the workplace is identified:* These procedures help ensure that chemically dependent employees receive effective treatment and rehabilitation. The procedures include these:
  - Documenting unacceptable behaviors by collecting specific information
  - Intervening with the identified employee
  - Referring the employee to a qualified resource for evaluation and treatment
  - Signing a return-to-work agreement
  - Following the specific continuing care plan
  - Monitoring the employee during early recovery

  If an employee refuses to follow the defined procedure (including evaluation) and the required treatment (if indicated), alternative actions must be specified in the policy document. Dismissal may be one of the actions.

- *Reporting requirements when the employee identified is a licensed professional such as a nurse or a physician:* Each facility's policy should reflect the requirements in its state. Some states, for example, have established programs that are authorized to assist chemically dependent nurses in lieu of reporting them for disciplinary action, others have memorandums of agreement with state peer assistance programs that defer reporting to the regulatory agency, and still other states require that nurses be reported to the state licensing agency whether or not they enter treatment. Most states have mandatory reporting laws, whether to the board of nursing or a designated alternative program. Therefore, the facility's task force should contact the state board of nursing prior to developing this portion of the fitness-for-duty policy.

- *Specific conditions and requirements when an employee returns to the workplace after treatment:* These may include the following:
  - A comprehensive evaluation of the employee's progress in treatment from the treatment provider

— A release from the treatment physician authorizing the
employee's return to the workplace

— A continuing care plan that specifies attendance at AA or NA,
nurse support group, and continuing care group meetings, as
well as restrictions or limitations on practice, including no
administration of mood-altering substances, specific shifts, and
specific nursing units

— A signed return-to-work agreement

All of these issues are covered in the sample policy and procedure document shown in figure 10-1. The sample document was developed for
use in a hospital, but it could easily be adapted to other health care
settings.

Drug-Testing Policy and Procedures

Within the past 5 to 10 years, employee drug testing has become a con-
troversial issue. In an attempt to detect drug usage in the workplace,
many employers have resorted to drug testing. Drug testing can be effective in identifying nurses who may be practicing under the influence
of mood-altering substances and can thereby promote both patient and
employee safety. Although testing is no panacea and its usefulness,
accuracy, and legality continue to be questioned, current trends indicate that more and more employers, including health care facilities,
are mandating drug testing for employees suspected of using drugs and
for applicants for employment.

Inclusion of a discussion of drug testing in this book does not imply
a blanket endorsement of its use. However, drug testing will be discussed as a tool that is available to health care facilities when used
appropriately as an adjunct to other documentation in encouraging
identified employees to accept help. Its use in obtaining information
on employees who may be actively using drugs or be chemically dependent in order to serve as grounds for dismissal, without first offering
treatment, is unacceptable. If a health care facility establishes drug-
testing policies and procedures, they should be part of a larger program
that encourages employees to seek treatment and supports their eventual return to work.

Drug testing is not the ultimate solution to the problem of alcohol or other drug use in the workplace, as many people assume. It con-
firms only one thing—that the specimen tested either contained or did
not contain mood-altering chemicals. If the test is done according to
acceptable standards and the specimen is not contaminated in any way,
the test can verify an employee's recent use of specific substances. The

test does not indicate that the employee is chemically dependent, nor does it suggest the level of impairment. Drug tests conducted under appropriate conditions and analyzed according to appropriate screening methods nonetheless provide an additional piece of documentation for use during interventions.

The task force responsible for developing an institution's drug-testing policies and procedures must be familiar with the provisions of the Americans with Disabilities Act to ensure that the facility meets the requirements of that law. The following guidelines can assist the task force in that effort:[2]

- The facility should demonstrate the need or "cause" for drug testing and be able to document a relationship between job performance and substance abuse. For example, a health care facility usually conducts drug tests because a nurse or another employee who is chemically dependent or using mood-altering chemicals in the workplace is jeopardizing patient safety and competent patient care. Random testing should be used only as part of a return-to-work agreement for recovering employees.
- The facility should develop drug-testing policies and procedures in consultation with all major employee groups in the health care facility, including union representatives, nursing, medical staff, security, human resources/personnel, laboratory, and legal counsel.
- The facility should use outside consultants to identify potential problems and assist in the development of a workable policy.
- The facility should modify employment contracts and union contracts to reflect the new policy.
- The facility should distribute copies of the policy to all staff.
- The facility should enforce the policy consistently.
- The facility should conduct drug tests carefully, following accepted procedures. The tests must be administered correctly and competently, following good analysis and chain-of-custody principles. The term *chain of custody* refers to procedures for ensuring that the specimens collected are not tampered with in any way. The process begins with collecting specimens in tamper-resistant containers and continues with appropriate labeling and documentation by everyone who handles the specimens until they are analyzed in the lab. The documentation serves as a paper trail of the custody of the sample at all times. Drug test results obtained when strict chain-of-custody procedures are not implemented can be legally challenged.
- When drug test results are positive, the facility should confirm them with an appropriate follow-up test.

- The facility should notify employees when drug test results are positive and inform them of the appeals process.
- The facility should keep the results confidential. Only staff with a need to know should be informed.
- The facility should establish a program to assist employees who are found to be chemically dependent.

A drug-testing policy (figure 10-2, for example) is one important step in developing an effective, legally sound drug-testing procedure. The facility's task force must also decide on the drug-testing method that will be used. Commonly accepted methods include thin-layer chromatography (TLC) and immunoassay techniques. Although one of the least expensive test methods, TLC is not as sensitive as

Figure 10-2. Sample Drug-Testing Policy

Objective

It is the intent of this policy to provide a drug-free, healthy, safe, and secure environment for both employees and patients.

Procedures

The hospital reserves the right to require drug and alcohol testing of any employee based on a "reasonable suspicion" that the employee has used alcohol or drugs and may be unfit for duty. "Reasonable suspicion" refers to a suspicion supported by documented, observed deficiencies in the employee's performance or behavior (see the fitness-for-duty policy).

1. The decision to conduct a drug test will be made by the employee's immediate supervisor and the department director.
2. A consent form for the drug test must be signed by the employee before the test is conducted.
3. The actual voiding and collection of all urine specimens shall be witnessed by the employee health nurse (or other identified individual). This procedure helps to ensure that specimens sent for analysis are in fact from the identified employee.
4. Each specimen will be coded with the employee's social security number to maintain confidentiality.
5. A strict chain of custody is to be maintained to ensure that specimens are not tampered with in any way. Specimens will be collected in tamper-resistant containers and a record will be maintained of every person who handles them from the time of collection until they are analyzed in the lab.
6. All drug-screening supplies, consents, security seals, and the like will be maintained by the employee health service.
7. All positive test results will be confirmed by a standard gas chromatography/mass spectrometry test. Test results will then be reported privately to the employee.
8. Employees whose test results are positive may request a retest. The second half of the original specimen, which is always kept in a secure place in the facility's laboratory, will be sent to the drug-testing laboratory for analysis.
9. An employee's refusal to cooperate or any attempt to invalidate or circumvent a drug test shall be considered sufficient cause for dismissal at any time.

immunoassay. Enzyme immunoassay and radioimmunoassay methods cost slightly more, but they are also more sensitive and more definitive. Whenever one of these methods produces a positive result, a more sophisticated technique, known as gas chromatography/mass spectrometry (GC/MS), should be used to confirm the finding.

Because alcohol is metabolized very quickly, a blood specimen should be taken whenever alcohol abuse is suspected. For other drugs, including prescription and illegal drugs, a urine specimen is usually effective.

In deciding which test method to use, the task force should consult with at least two or three reputable independent laboratories experienced in providing comprehensive and confidential drug testing. The health care institution's own laboratory personnel can recommend independent facilities in the area. As the task force consults with these laboratories, it will also be evaluating them with a view to selecting one to conduct the institution's drug tests. Once a laboratory is chosen, laboratory staff should train selected hospital personnel in how to collect samples and interpret test results.

Education and Training

After all policies governing alcohol or drug use in the workplace have been approved by the administration, the next step is to disseminate them to employees and implement a facilitywide educational program. Every member of the staff, from top-level managers to entry-level employees, needs to understand chemical dependency issues and policies. Without a strong ongoing educational effort, the most comprehensive policies and procedures will fail or, at best, fall far short of success.

Education on the key facts of chemical dependency and the institution's process for assisting affected employees will equip staff with the knowledge necessary to get help for themselves and others. It can also help them overcome prejudices, fears, and misconceptions, thus setting the stage for a major change in attitudes and behaviors. These two educational goals, in turn, contribute significantly to the new program's success.

Two separate programs, one for all staff and the other for managers, can be offered. Ideally, an educator or practitioner in the field of chemical dependency who understands the dynamics of the disease, the effects of alcohol or drug use in the workplace, and management principles and responsibilities should conduct the programs. If the facility has an EAP counselor who is skilled in leading educational sessions and is up-to-date on chemical dependency issues, he or she could also be qualified to carry out the educational program.

Education for All Staff

All employees of the health care facility, both staff and management, should receive education in the following areas:

- The effects of mood-altering chemicals, such as alcohol and other drugs, in the workplace
  - Specific drug classifications
  - Signs and symptoms
  - How job performance is impaired
- The nature of chemical dependency
  - Loss of control
  - Compulsive use
  - Continued use despite negative consequences
  - Denial, including minimization, rationalization, and projection
- Obstacles to getting help
  - Attitudes of society toward chemical dependency
  - Attitudes among health care professionals and workers
  - Enabling
- The facility's policies and procedures regarding employee alcohol or other drug use
  - Fitness for duty
  - Drug screening
  - Support for treatment
  - Return to work
  - Consequences for noncompliance
- The responsibility of all employees to promote a drug-free workplace
- Resources for assistance and how to use them
  - Employee assistance program
  - Human resources department
  - Supervisor or director
  - Psychiatric nurse liaison
- Methods for supporting chemically dependent employees while they are in treatment and when they return to the workplace

Additional Education for Nurses

The educational session for all nurses (including managers) should also cover some issues specific to the nursing profession, such as the following:

- How nursing practice is impaired
- The high-risk nature of nursing
  - Attitudes
  - Beliefs
  - Access to drugs
  - High-stress environment
  - Unrealistic expectations of themselves
- Drug diversion
  - Signs of diversion
  - Failure to follow drug policies and procedures
- Nursing practice act
  - Violations
  - Responsibilities of each licensee
  - Reporting requirements
- Limitations or restrictions on practice when recovering nurses return to the workplace after treatment and accommodations mandated by the Americans with Disabilities Act

Education for Managers

In addition to the all-staff educational program, managers require specific education and training in a number of areas:

- What part the manager or supervisor plays in the identification, intervention, and return to work of chemically dependent employees
- How to gather specific information on an employee suspected of using drugs
  - Observations by manager
  - Verification of observations by another manager
  - Co-workers' reports
  - Written information or reports prepared by the suspected employee
  - Employee records: attendance reports, performance evaluations, incident reports
- How to confront the employee with evidence of chemical dependency
  - Preparation for the intervention
  - Specific steps in conducting an intervention
  - Handling of employee objections during the intervention or noncompliance with the intervention team's recommendations
- How to get appropriate help for the employee
  - Available resources

  −Treatment programs
- How to effectively inform co-workers
  −Information to be shared
  −Informational meeting with co-workers
- How to facilitate the employee's return to the workplace
  −Communication with the employee while he or she is still in treatment
  −Participation in discharge planning: determining whether the employee is ready to return to the job and whether there should be any limitations or restrictions when the employee returns to work
- How to conduct a return-to-work meeting
  −Participants
  −Specific questions and issues to address
  −Return-to-work agreement
- How to evaluate and supervise the recovering employee
  −Monitoring of compliance with the return-to-work agreement
  −Evaluation of job performance
  −Recognition of the signs of relapse
- What to do if the recovering employee relapses

Nurse managers should also receive specific training in:

- How to detect drug diversion
- How to determine where the nurse should return to practice
- How to prepare the workplace for restrictions or limitations on the nurse's practice regarding controlled drug administration, shifts, and supervision

In addition, the educational program for managers should include skill-training sessions. Through such techniques as role-playing, demonstrations, and case studies, managers have an opportunity to develop their intervention, documentation, and other skills.

Resources

In developing alcohol and drug abuse policies and procedures, as well as the staff educational programs that follow, health care facilities can tap a number of state, local, and in-house resources. Resources include the facility's own employee assistance program (EAP), psychiatric nurse liaisons, monitors for recovering nurses, the state board of nursing, local chemical dependency treatment programs and support groups, as well as chemical dependency consultants. Nurse managers and other supervisors in the facility can also consult these resources when they suspect an employee of using drugs, are arranging an intervention, planning an employee's return to work, or concerned about a possible relapse.

Employee Assistance Programs

Some health care facilities maintain EAPs to assist employees experiencing personal difficulties. Employees who use EAP services usually have problems with alcohol or other drugs, personal finances, family relationships, legal issues, or emotions and stress, which may or may not be interfering with their job performance. The purpose of the EAP is to help identify and then resolve these problems and maintain confidentiality throughout.

Employees often seek out EAP services directly. Managers or supervisors may also refer employees to EAPs. Effective EAPs usually educate both staff and supervisors about their services and how to use them. EAP counselors also serve as consultants to supervisors when employee job performance is being affected. In these ways, EAPs contribute to positive labor–management relations, problem resolution, and the employee's dignity.

There are two basic types of EAPs: internal and external. Internal programs are established and staffed by the health care facility and usually come under the direction of the human resources department. External programs provide services to the facility on a contract basis. Facilities that do not currently have EAPs and would like to provide EAP services to employees can contact the Employee Assistance Professionals Association in Arlington, Virginia, which can supply resource materials.

Psychiatric Nurse Liaisons

Many hospitals employ psychiatric nurse clinicians to provide a number of consultation services to staff. Their main role is to assist staff in meeting the mental health needs of patients. In health care facilities that do not have a formal EAP, these clinicians may also function as consultants to nursing administration on job performance, chemical dependency, and mental health issues affecting nurses. In some cases, these clinicians may also consult with all managers, as needed, not just nursing.

Nurse clinicians who have specific expertise and experience with chemically dependent individuals can serve as an important resource when nurse managers need advice on managing chemically dependent nurses. Otherwise, managers will probably obtain more valuable assistance from other resources.

Monitors for Recovering Nurses and Other Staff

After recovering nurses return to work, their nurse managers may need or want to consult with the people responsible for monitoring the nurses' recovery progress and compliance with the return-to-work agreement. The monitor is usually a nurse designated by nursing administration, an EAP counselor, a psychiatric nurse liaison, or an employee health nurse. The nurse manager never serves as a monitor; his or her role is to supervise.

In many ways, monitors function as case managers, facilitating effective communication among nurse managers, continuing care counselors, nurse support group facilitators, and recovering nurses. They collect and review reports from continuing care counselors and nurse support group facilitators, as well as forms that nurses must submit verifying attendance at support group meetings. They also coordinate periodic meetings to review nurses' recovery progress, discuss problem areas, and recommend solutions. Because monitors are invariably knowledgeable about the disease of chemical dependency and the recovery process, they can be a valuable resource on return-to-work issues such as relapse.

State Boards of Nursing

All nurse managers should be familiar with state statutes pertaining to the practice of nursing. These statutes, usually referred to as nursing practice acts, explain how to verify a nurse's current licensure status; violations, including impaired practice, use of controlled drugs, and arrests for using illegal, addictive drugs; and employers' responsibilities for reporting violations to the board or other licensing and regulatory agency. Many state boards provide education and consultation services to health care facilities that request them. Boards of nursing can be a useful resource for hiring nurses or gathering data on troubled nurses prior to an intervention.

Alternative, Diversion, and Peer Assistance Programs

Alternative, diversion, and peer assistance programs have been developed by states and nurses' associations to help chemically dependent nurses obtain the appropriate level of treatment and return to practice after being stabilized. Programs established by state legislation to provide services, in lieu of disciplinary action, to nurses who violate the nursing practice act are usually known as alternative or diversion programs. Nurses' participation in these programs may or may not be voluntary. Voluntary programs operated by nurses' associations are known as peer assistance programs. In general, both program types can provide some educational and consultation services to health care employers.

To determine whether such programs exist in the facility's state, and what services they offer, a representative of the facility can contact both the state nursing board and the state nurses' association. The nursing board or nurses' association should also be able to supply information on support groups specifically designed for recovering nurses. In addition, nurses' associations sometimes hold workshops and seminars on techniques for identifying and managing chemically dependent nurses.

Support Groups

Support groups available to nurses and other health care professionals include Alcoholics Anonymous (AA), Narcotics Anonymous (NA), and various professional support groups. Lists of local resources are available from telephone directories, chemical dependency treatment centers, alcoholism and drug addiction agencies, social service agencies, and religious institutions. Because AA groups are widespread, even in geographic areas with very few alcoholics, it is relatively easy to find an AA group nearby. The AA group, in turn, can often provide information about other support groups in the area.

Chemical Dependency Treatment Programs

Chemical dependency treatment programs provide various levels of treatment, and staff may or may not be experienced in working specifically with nurses and other health care professionals. (Chapter 6 discussed the criteria for selecting a chemical dependency treatment program.) Once a facility has located one or two programs that meet most of the criteria, nurse managers will be able to tap the considerable expertise of program staff. Program staff can usually provide assistance and advice on a wide range of issues related to chemical dependency in the workplace. They might even be enlisted to conduct educational programs for health care facility employees.

Consultants

Consultants in the chemical dependency field can be helpful when nursing administration, or the facility as a whole, decides to establish a program to assist nurses. Consultants help set up the programs, train in-house staff to run them, and then leave. Skilled consultants can advise facilities on labor–management issues, policy issues and formulation, legal precautions, employee benefits, and other important considerations. Some consultants are also qualified to conduct educational programs on chemical dependency for staff and managers.

When choosing a consultant, health care facilities should contact state nurses' associations, state boards of nursing, local drug and alcohol agencies, and other health care facilities that have used consultants to establish chemical dependency programs. Local and state hospital associations, as well as the American Hospital Association, can usually supply the names of facilities that have developed effective programs.

The use of alcohol and other drugs in the workplace and the resulting impairment of job performance are significant problems in health care facilities. The solution, as outlined in this chapter, requires a multidimensional approach comprising strong policies and procedures, effective staff education, and access to skilled resources.

Summary

The process outlined in this book for assisting chemically dependent nurses has the best chance of succeeding when the health care facility applies it to all employees, not just nurses. To establish a facilitywide program, a task force representing all major staff groups should be formed.

The task force's primary charge should be to develop clear, comprehensive policies and procedures that encourage consistent management of chemically dependent employees. To guide policy development, task force members first need to agree on an institutional philosophy. A good philosophy usually reaffirms the facility's responsibility for providing a drug-free workplace, and appropriate intervention and treatment services for those employees who are impaired.

Once the philosophy statement has been approved by administration, the task force is ready to draft a fitness-for-duty policy. This policy spells out the facility's expectations of employees, supervisors' responsibilities when employees violate policy, treatment and other support services, and conditions on which recovering employees may return to work.

Administration may also charge the task force with designing a drug-testing policy and program. Used appropriately, drug tests can provide another piece of information for managers to use in encouraging chemically dependent employees to seek help. They should not be used solely to gather evidence for dismissal without offering employees treatment.

When the new policies have been approved by administration, copies should be distributed to every employee. All staff, from administrators to entry-level employees, should also receive education on chemical dependency issues and policies. Without a strong ongoing educational effort, the most comprehensive policies and procedures will fall short of success.

In developing alcohol and drug abuse policies and procedures, as well as the staff educational programs to follow, health care facilities can tap a number of state, local, and in-house resources. These include the facility's own employee assistance program, the state board of nursing, local chemical dependency treatment programs and support groups, as well as chemical dependency consultants.

☐ *References*

1. National Institute on Drug Abuse. *Drug Abuse in the Workplace.* Washington, DC: Department of Health and Human Services, 1986.
2. Dogoloff, L. I., and Angarola, R. T. *Urine Testing in the Workplace.* Rockville, MD: American Council for Drug Education, 1985.

Afterword

T. M.
J. B.
R. T.
M. Mc.
T. B.

These are the initials of nurses who died during the time it took me to write this book. Cause of death — chemical dependency. The details surrounding their deaths share some common circumstances: they were working as nurses until the time of their deaths, their colleagues were concerned about them and shocked by their deaths but unaware of the extent of their problems, and the procedures outlined in this book were not known or used by their supervisors.

I knew none of the nurses personally. Their deaths came to my attention through communications with others who work with and care about chemically dependent nurses. Yet their deaths seem to me so sad and so senseless. Because I have seen how effective the process discussed in this book can be, it is easy at times to be lulled into the illusion that this is the way all chemically dependent nurses are helped. But this is not so — at least not yet.

We must never forget that chemical dependency kills! Although we as nurses have become more educated and skilled in various aspects of nursing, many nurse managers need guidance, support, and education before they will be equipped to take appropriate action, without delay, when a nurse exhibits signs and symptoms of chemical dependency. As Thomas Huxley so aptly once said, "Perhaps the most valuable result of all education is the ability to make yourself do the thing you have to do, when it ought to be done, whether you like it or not. It is the first lesson that ought to be learned."

This book represents the first step in the educational process. After reading it, nurse managers should be able to:

- Understand the nature of chemical dependency
- Accept their role in intervening with chemically dependent nurses and actively assisting them without delay to prevent the continuing advance of the disease and its accompanying dysfunction
- Implement a realistic, effective model that comprehensively addresses the needs of chemically dependent nurses and the health care workplace
- Accept their key role and responsibility in influencing and implementing effective chemical dependency policies and procedures in their institutions

In meeting these objectives, this book will have also achieved its primary goals, namely, to help nurses suffering from the disease of chemical dependency get treatment, get well, and recover and to empower nurse managers to manage chemically dependent nurses in a way that benefits both the nurses and the workplace.

A key point made throughout this book has been that chemical dependency is a cunning and baffling disease characterized by denial and a firmly entrenched delusional system. The denial and delusion prevent nurses from realizing that they have a problem and keep them from seeking help. Through their understanding of the nature of chemical dependency, nurse managers can actively intervene. They simply cannot wait for a nurse to ask for help, because it is very unlikely that a chemically dependent nurse would be able to ask for help.

As chapter 4 pointed out, enabling is perhaps the most significant obstacle to getting help for the nurse who is experiencing problems. No matter how well intentioned the nurse manager is or how much he or she cares about the nurse, if the manager's actions in any way prevent the nurse from feeling the consequences of his or her use of alcohol or other drugs, the manager is enabling that nurse to continue in the destructive, progressive spiral characteristic of chemical dependency. Effective confrontation through an intervention most significantly makes the nurse feel the consequence of his or her chemical use. If a nurse manager's own denial is not pierced by education and acceptance of the disease, he or she will be unable to effectively intervene with the nurse. Acceptance of the premise that chemical dependency can affect anyone, regardless of their profession, is the first step that must be taken.

The next step is to develop the skills necessary to effectively identify and intervene with chemically dependent nurses. Active intervention involves learning how to:

- Identify the chemically dependent nurse through signs and
  symptoms
- Prepare for and conduct an intervention
- Consult with treatment providers on treatment and continuing
  care issues
- Assist the nurse in returning to the workplace after treatment
- Supervise the recovering nurse
- Promote the development and implementation of policies and
  procedures for the workplace that pertain to alcohol and other
  drug use
- Gather support for and spearhead the development of a
  facilitywide program to assist chemically dependent employees
  in getting treatment, returning to work, and recovering from their
  disease

The overwhelming problems — for the nurse and the workplace —
that result from active, untreated chemical dependency must be
stopped. Perpetuating the dysfunction caused by the disease must end.
The process for assisting chemically dependent nurses described in this
book is not a theory or a proposal but a step-by-step process that has
been successfully implemented in hospitals and other health care facilities around the country.

My hope is that the guidelines presented in *Managing the Chemically Dependent Nurse* will help nurse managers in their efforts to help
other nurses; to interrupt the progression of a devastating, chronic disease; and to set the recovery process in motion. It is truly a win–win
situation: the nurse wins because his or her recovery was made possible, and the nurse manager wins because she or he cared enough to
do what is necessary and right. It can be a transforming experience
for everyone involved: the chemically dependent nurse, the nurse
manager, the nurse's co-workers, and the institution.

Suggested Resources

Books

Alcoholics Anonymous. New York City: Alcoholics Anonymous World Services, Inc., 1976.

American Hospital Association, Office of Regulatory Affairs. *Americans with Disabilities Act: A Practical Guide for Hospitals.* Legal memorandum no. 15. Chicago: AHA, Feb. 1991.

Crosby, L. R., and Bissell, L. *To Care Enough.* Minneapolis: Johnson Institute, 1989.

Dogoloff, L. I., and Angarola, R. T. *Urine Testing in the Workplace.* Rockville, MD: American Council on Drug Education, 1985.

Fitzgerald, K. W. *Alcoholism: The Genetic Inheritance.* New York City: Doubleday, 1988.

Gorski, T. T., and Miller, M. *Counseling for Relapse Prevention.* Independence, MO: Herald House-Independence Press, 1982.

Johnson, V. E. *Intervention: How to Help Someone Who Doesn't Want Help.* Minneapolis: Johnson Institute, 1986.

Meryman, R. *Broken Promises, Mended Dreams.* New York City: Berkley Books, 1984.

Milan, J. R., and Ketchem, K. *Under the Influence.* Seattle: Madrona Publishers, 1981.

National Institute on Drug Abuse. *Drug Abuse in the Workplace.* DHHS Publication no. (ADM) 86-1477. Rockville, MD: NIDA, 1986.

Sullivan, E., Bissell, L., and Williams, E. *Chemical Dependency in Nursing: The Deadly Diversion.*, Menlo Park, CA: Addison-Wesley Publishing, 1988.

Twerski, A. *It Happens to Doctors Too.* Center City, MN: Hazelden, 1982.

Videos

The Substance-Abusing Nurse, 1991
American Hospital Association Services, Inc.
P.O. Box 99376
Chicago, IL 60693
(800/242-2626)

Care for the Caregiver, 1989
Intervention Project for Nurses
1200 Gulf Life Drive, Suite 915
Jacksonville, FL 32207
(904/348-2720)

Enabling: Masking Reality, 1989
Intervention: Facing Reality, 1989
Johnson Institute
7151 Metro Boulevard
Minneapolis, MN 55435
(800/231-5165)

Professional Associations for Chemical Dependency Nursing

Drug and Alcohol Nursing Association (DANA)
113 W. Franklin Street
Baltimore, MD 21201
(301/752-3318)

National Consortium on Chemical Dependency Nursing (NCCDN)
975 Oak Street, Suite 675
Eugene, OR 97401
(800/876-2236)

National Nurses Society on Addictions (NNSA)
5700 Old Orchard Road
Skokie, IL 60077
(708/966-5010)

Support Groups for Professionals

Anesthetists in Recovery (AIR)
American Association of Nurse Anesthetists
216 Higgins Road
Park Ridge, IL 60068
(In Illinois: 800/433-3786; outside Illinois: 800/654-5167)

International Nurses Anonymous
1020 Sunset Drive
Lawrence, KS 66044
(913/842-3893)
(Open to nurses who are in personal recovery or who are members of Al-Anon)